This report contains the collective views of an international group of experts and does not necessarily represent the decisions or the stated policy of the United Nations Environment Programme, the International Labour Organisation, or the World Health Organization

Environmental Health Criteria 98

TETRAMETHRIN

Published under the joint sponsorship of the United Nations Environment Programme, the International Labour Organisation, and the World Health Organization

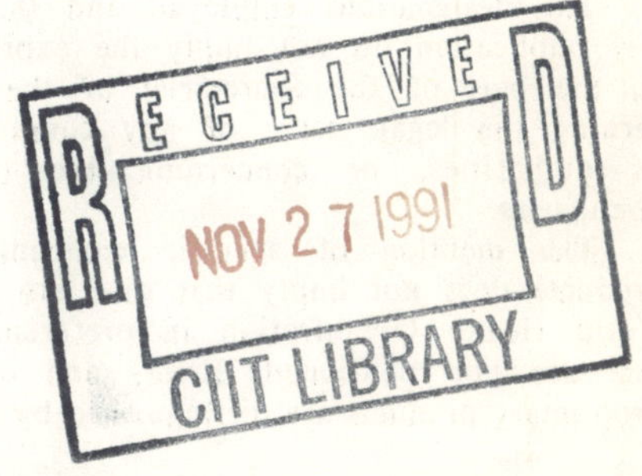

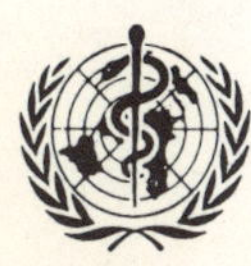

World Health Organization
Geneva, 1990

The **International Programme on Chemical Safety (IPCS)** is a joint venture of the United Nations Environment Programme, the International Labour Organisation, and the World Health Organization. The main objective of the IPCS is to carry out and disseminate evaluations of the effects of chemicals on human health and the quality of the environment. Supporting activities include the development of epidemiological, experimental laboratory, and risk-assessment methods that could produce internationally comparable results, and the development of manpower in the field of toxicology. Other activities carried out by the IPCS include the development of know-how for coping with chemical accidents, coordination of laboratory testing and epidemiological studies, and promotion of research on the mechanisms of the biological action of chemicals.

WHO Library Cataloguing in Publication Data

Tetramethrin.

(Environmental health criteria ; 98)

1. Pyrethrins I. Series

ISBN 92 4 154298 5 (NLM Classification: WA 240)
ISSN 0250-863X

Printed in Finland

DHSS — Vammala — 5000

CONTENTS

ENVIRONMENTAL HEALTH CRITERIA FOR TETRAMETHRIN

INTRODUCTION 11

1. SUMMARY, EVALUATION, CONCLUSIONS, AND RECOMMENDATIONS 14

1.1 Summary and evaluation 14
1.1.1 Identity, physical and chemical properties, analytical methods 14
1.1.2 Production and use 14
1.1.3 Human exposure 15
1.1.4 Environmental exposure and fate 15
1.1.5 Uptake, metabolism, and excretion 15
1.1.6 Effects on organisms in the environment 16
1.1.7 Effects on experimental animals and *in vitro* test systems 16
1.1.8 Effects on human beings 18
1.2 Conclusions 18
1.3 Recommendations 19

2. IDENTITY, PHYSICAL AND CHEMICAL PROPERTIES, ANALYTICAL METHODS 20

2.1 Identity 20
2.2 Physical and chemical properties 21
2.3 Analytical methods 21

3. SOURCES AND LEVELS OF HUMAN AND ENVIRONMENTAL EXPOSURE 25

3.1 Industrial production 25
3.2 Use patterns 25
3.3 Residues in food 25
3.4 Exposure levels from household use 25
3.5 Environment levels 25

4. ENVIRONMENTAL TRANSPORT, DISTRIBUTION, AND TRANSFORMATION 26

4.1 Abiotic degradation in air and water 26

5. KINETICS AND METABOLISM 28

5.1 Metabolism in mammals 28
5.2 Enzymatic systems for biotransformation 31

6. EFFECTS ON ORGANISMS IN THE ENVIRONMENT 32

6.1 Aquatic organisms 32
6.2 Terrestrial organisms 32

7. EFFECTS ON EXPERIMENTAL ANIMALS AND *IN VITRO* TEST SYSTEMS 34

7.1 Single exposures 34
7.2 Irritation and sensitization 35
7.2.1 Eye irritation 35
7.2.2 Skin irritation 36
7.2.3 Sensitization 36
7.3 Short-term exposure studies 36
7.3.1 Oral 36
7.3.2 Inhalation 38
7.4 Long-term exposures and carcinogenicity 38
7.5 Mutagenicity 40
7.6 Reproduction, embryotoxicity, and teratogenicity 40
7.7 Neurotoxicity - mode of action 45

8. EFFECTS ON HUMANS 47

9. PREVIOUS EVALUATIONS BY INTERNATIONAL BODIES 48

REFERENCES 49

APPENDIX I 56

FRENCH TRANSLATION OF SUMMARY, EVALUATION, CONCLUSIONS, AND RECOMMENDATIONS 63

WHO TASK GROUP ON ENVIRONMENTAL HEALTH CRITERIA FOR TETRAMETHRIN

Members

Dr V. Benes, Toxicology and Reference Laboratory, Institute of Hygiene and Epidemiology, Prague, Czechoslovakia

Dr A.J. Browning, Toxicology Evaluation Section, Department of Community Services and Health, Woden, ACT, Australia

Dr S. Dobson, Institute of Terrestrial Ecology, Monks Wood Experimental Station, Abbots Ripton, Huntingdon, United Kingdom *(Chairman)*

Dr P. Hurley, Office of Pesticide Programme, US Environmental Protection Agency, Washington DC, USA

Dr K. Imaida, Section of Tumor Pathology, Division of Pathology, National Institute of Hygienic Sciences, Setagaya-Ku, Tokyo, Japan

Dr S.K. Kashyap, National Institute of Occupational Health, (I.C.M.R.) Ahmedabad, India *(Vice-Chairman)*

Dr Yu. I. Kundiev, Research Institute of Labour, Hygiene and Occupational Diseases, Ul. Saksaganskogo, Kiev, USSR

Dr J.P. Leahey, ICI Agrochemicals, Jealotts Hill Research Station, Bracknell, United Kingdom *(Rapporteur)*

Dr M. Matsuo, Sumitomo Chemical Company, Biochemistry and Toxicology Laboratory, Kasugade-naka, Konohana-Ku, Osaka, Japan

Dr J. Sekizawa, Division of Information on Chemical Safety, National Institute of Hygienic Sciences, Setagaya-Ku, Tokyo, Japan *(Rapporteur)*

Representatives of Other Organization

Mr M. L'Hotellier, Groupement International des Associations Nationales de Fabricants de Produits Agrochimiques (GIFAP)

Dr N. Punja, Groupement International des Associations Nationales de Fabricants de Produits Agrochimiques (GIFAP)

Secretariat

Dr K.W. Jager, International Programme on Chemical Safety, World Health Organization, Geneva, Switzerland *(Secretary)*

Dr R. Plestina, Division of Vector Biology and Control, World Health Organization, Geneva, Switzerland

NOTE TO READERS OF THE CRITERIA DOCUMENTS

Every effort has been made to present information in the criteria documents as accurately as possible without unduly delaying their publication. In the interest of all users of the environmental health criteria documents, readers are kindly requested to communicate any errors that may have occurred to the Manager of the International Programme on Chemical Safety, World Health Organization, Geneva, Switzerland, in order that they may be included in corrigenda, which will appear in subsequent volumes.

* * *

A detailed data profile and a legal file can be obtained from the International Register of Potentially Toxic Chemicals, Palais des Nations, 1211 Geneva 10, Switzerland (Telephone No. 7988400 - 7985850).

* * *

The proprietary information contained in this document cannot replace documentation for registration purposes, because the latter has to be closely linked to the source, the manufacturing route, and the purity/impurities of the substance to be registered. The data should be used in accordance with paragraphs 82-84 and recommendations paragraph 90 of the Second FAO Government Consultation [5].

ENVIRONMENTAL HEALTH CRITERIA FOR TETRAMETHRIN

A WHO Task Group on Environmental Health Criteria for Tetramethrin met in Geneva from 24 to 28 October 1988. Dr M. Mercier, Manager, IPCS, opened the meeting and welcomed the participants on behalf of the three IPCS cooperrating organizations (UNEP/ILO/WHO). The group reviewed and revised the draft monograph and made an evaluation of the risks for human health and the environment from exposure to tetramethrin.

The first draft was prepared by DR J. MIYAMOTO and DR M. MATSUO of Sumitomo Chemical Company, and DR J. SEKIZAWA of the National Institute of Hygienic Sciences, Tokyo, Japan.

The second draft was prepared by the IPCS secretariat, incorporating comments received following circulation of the first draft to the IPCS contact points for Environmental Health Criteria documents. Dr K.W. Jager and Dr P.G. Jenkins, both members of the IPCS Central Unit, were responsible for the technical development and editing, respectively, of this monograph.

The assistance of the Sumitomo Chemical Company in making available to the IPCS and the Task Group its toxicological proprietary information on tetramethrin is gratefully acknowledged. This allowed the Task Group to make its evaluation on the basis of more complete data.

* * *

The United Kingdom Department of Health and Social Security generously supported the cost of printing.

ABBREVIATIONS

CA	chrysanthemic acid
FID-GC	gas chromatography with flame ionization detector
HPI	cyclohexane-1,2-dicarboximide
HPLC	high performance liquid chromatography
HPTLC	high performance thin-layer chromatography
ip	intraperitoneal
MTI	*N*-(hydroxymethyl)-3,4,5,6-tetrahydrophthalamide
NOEL	no-observed-effect level
TLC	thin-layer chromatography
TPI	3,4,5,6-tetrahydrophthalimide
TPIA	3,4,5,6-tetrahydrophthalic acid

INTRODUCTION

SYNTHETIC PYRETHROIDS - A PROFILE

1. During investigations to modify the chemical structures of natural pyrethrins, a certain number of synthetic pyrethroids were produced with improved physical and chemical properties and greater biological activity. Several of the earlier synthetic pyrethroids were successfully commercialized, mainly for the control of household insects. Other more recent pyrethroids have been introduced as agricultural insecticides because of their excellent activity against a wide range of insect pests and their non-persistence in the environment.

2. The pyrethroids constitute another group of insecticides in addition to organochlorine, organophosphorus, carbamate, and other compounds. Pyrethroids commercially available to date include allethrin, resmethrin, d-phenothrin, and tetramethrin (for insects of public health importance), and cypermethrin, deltamethrin, fenvalerate, and permethrin (mainly for agricultural insects). Other pyrethroids are also available including furamethrin, kadethrin, and tellallethrin (usually for household insects), fenpropathrin, tralomethrin, cyhalothrin, lambda-cyhalothrin, tefluthrin, cyfluthrin, flucythrinate, fluvalinate, and biphenate (for agricultural insects).

3. Toxicological evaluations of several synthetic pyrethroids have been performed by the FAO/WHO Joint Meeting on Pesticide Residues (JMPR). The acceptable daily intake (ADI) has been estimated by the JMPR for cypermethrin, deltamethrin, fenvalerate, permethrin, d-phenothrin, cyfluthrin, cyhalothrin, and flucythrinate.

4. Chemically, synthetic pyrethroids are esters of specific acids (e.g., chrysanthemic acid, halo-substituted chrysanthemic acid, 2-(4-chlorophenyl)-3-methylbutyric acid) and alcohols (e.g., allethrolone, 3-phenoxybenzyl alcohol). For certain pyrethroids, the

asymmetric centre(s) exist in the acid and/or alcohol moiety, and the commercial products sometimes consist of a mixture of both optical (1R/1S or d/l) and geometric (cis/trans) isomers. However, most of the insecticidal activity of such products may reside in only one or two isomers. Some of the products (e.g., d-phenothrin, deltamethrin) consist only of such active isomer(s).

5. Synthetic pyrethroids are neuropoisons acting on the axons in the peripheral and central nervous systems by interacting with sodium channels in mammals and/or insects. A single dose produces toxic signs in mammals, such as tremors, hyperexcitability, salivation, choreoathetosis, and paralysis. The signs disappear fairly rapidly, and the animals recover, generally within a week. At near-lethal dose levels, synthetic pyrethroids cause transient changes in the nervous system, such as axonal swelling and/or breaks and myelin degeneration in sciatic nerves. They are not considered to cause delayed neurotoxicity of the kind induced by some organophosphorus compounds. The mechanism of toxicity of synthetic pyrethroids and their classification into two types are discussed in the Appendix.

6. Some pyrethroids (e.g., deltamethrin, fenvalerate, cyhalothrin, lambda-cyhalothrin, flucythrinate, and cypermethrin) may cause a transient itching and/or burning sensation in exposed human skin.

7. Synthetic pyrethroids are generally metabolized in mammals through ester hydrolysis, oxidation, and conjugation, and there is no tendency to accumulate in tissues. In the environment, synthetic pyrethroids are fairly rapidly degraded in soil and in plants. Ester hydrolysis and oxidation at various sites on the molecule are the major degradation processes. The pyrethroids are strongly adsorbed on soil and sediments, and hardly eluted with water. There is little tendency for bioaccumulation in organisms.

8. Because of low application rates and rapid degradation in the environment, residues in food are generally low.

9. Synthetic pyrethroids have been shown to be toxic for fish, aquatic arthropods, and honey-bees in laboratory tests. But, in practical usage, no serious adverse effects have been noticed because of the low rates of application and lack of persistence in the environment. The toxicity of synthetic pyrethroids in birds and domestic animals is low.

10. In addition to the evaluation documents of FAO/WHO, there are several good reviews and books on the chemistry, metabolism, mammalian toxicity, environmental effects, etc. of synthetic pyrethroids, including those by Elliott [3], Miyamoto [34], Miyamoto & Kearney [35], and Leahey [26].

1. SUMMARY, EVALUATION, CONCLUSIONS, AND RECOMMENDATIONS

1.1 Summary and Evaluation

1.1.1 Identity, physical and chemical properties, analytical methods

Tetramethrin was first synthesized in 1964 and first marketed in 1965. Chemically, it is an ester of chrysanthemic acid (2,2-dimethyl-3-(2,2-dimethylvinyl)-cyclopropanecarboxylic acid) with 3,4,5,6-tetrahydrophthalimidomethyl alcohol. It is a mixture of four stereoisomers: [1R,trans], [1R,cis], [1S,trans], and [1S,cis]. In technical products, the composition ratio of the isomers is roughly 4:1:4:1. Among the isomers, the [1R,trans] isomer is the most active biologically followed by the [1R,cis] isomer. A mixture of the [1R,cis] and [1R,trans] isomers (1:4) is commercialized under the trade name of 'Neo-Pynamin Forte' (designated as 1R,*cis/trans*-tetramethrin in this monograph).

Technical grade tetramethrin is a colourless solid with a melting point of 65-80°C. The specific gravity is 1.11 at 20 °C, and the vapour pressure is 0.946 mPa (7.1 x 10^{-6} mmHg) at 30 °C. It is sparingly soluble in water (4.6 mg/litre at 30 °C) but soluble in organic solvents such as hexane, methanol, and xylene. It is stable to heat but unstable to light and air. The [1R,cis/trans] isomer of tetramethrin is a yellow viscous liquid but otherwise has physical and chemical properties similar to tetramethrin.

Residue analysis is carried out by quantification using dual-wavelength densitometry (370-230 nm). Gas chromatography with flame ionization detector is used for technical product analysis. Formulation analysis can be carried out by high-performance liquid chromatography with an infra-red detector.

1.1.2 Production and use

The annual world-wide production of tetramethrin is estimated to be a few hundred tonnes. It is mostly used for indoor pest control, formulated as an aerosol, an emulsifiable concentrate, or a mosquito coil. Formulations in combination with other insecticides and synergists are also prepared.

1.1.3 Human exposure

The general population may be exposed to tetramethrin primarily through its use in indoor pest control. When tetramethrin is used as recommended, the aerial levels and those of its 1R isomer are unlikely to exceed 0.5 mg/m^3, and the compound will degrade rapidly. Therefore, the exposure of the general population is expected to be very low. Tetramethrin is not used on food crops.

1.1.4 Environmental exposure and fate

Rapid degradation occurs when a thin film of tetramethrin is exposed to sunlight. The major photoreactions during a 2-h exposure (30% conversion) were: epoxidation at the isobutenyl double bond; oxidation at the *trans*-methyl of the isobutenyl group to hydroxymethyl, aldehyde, and carboxylic acid; and hydroperoxidation to allylic hydroperoxide.

No data are available on the exact levels of tetramethrin in the environment, but with the current domestic pattern of use and when tetramethrin is used as recommended, environmental exposure is expected to be very low. Degradation to less toxic products is rapid.

1.1.5 Uptake, metabolism, and excretion

In rats, tetramethrin radiolabelled in the acid or alcohol moiety is readily taken up, metabolized, and excreted after oral or subcutaneous administration. Approximately 95% is excreted in 5-7 days in the urine and faeces in more or less equal amounts. The tissue residues from both administration routes are very low. The metabolic reactions are: ester cleavage; loss of the hydroxymethyl group from the alcohol moiety; reduction of the 1-2 bond of the alcohol moiety; oxidation at the isobutenyl methyl moiety of the acid and at the 2-, 3-, and 4-positions of the alcohol moiety; conjugation of the resultant acids and alcohols with glucuronic acid; and cis/trans isomerization.

1.1.6 Effects on organisms in the environment

Only very limited information is available. Tetramethrin is highly toxic for fish, the 96-h LC_{50} values for two species being 19 and 21 μg/litre. A third species showed a 48-h LC_{50} of 200 μg/litre and a no-observed-effect level of 50 μg/litre. The no-observed-effect level for Daphnia is 50 μg/litre. Tetramethrin has very low toxicity to birds but is toxic for honey bees. Because tetramethrin is rapidly degraded, and provided its use is limited to buildings, as recommended, the potential that it has for producing effects on the environment is unlikely to be realised.

1.1.7 Effects on experimental animals and *in vitro* test systems

The acute oral toxicity of tetramethrin is low. The LD_{50} for rats is >5000 mg/kg with both the racemic mixture and the 1R, cis/trans isomer, whereas for mice it is about 2000 mg/kg (racemate) and 1060 mg/kg (1R, cis/trans). The acute dermal toxicities in both rat and mouse, as well as in the rabbit, are also low; the LD_{50} in rats and mice is >5000 mg/kg, while in rabbits it is >2000 mg/kg (all studies were done with racemic mixture). In acute inhalation studies, the LC_{50} in rats and mice was 2500 mg/m^3 for the racemic mixture and >1180 mg/m^3 for the 1R, cis/trans isomer. The toxic signs include hyperexcitability, tremor, ataxia, and depression (general signs combined from all the acute studies). Mice were somewhat more susceptible than rats, but no differences were observed in susceptibility between males and females. Tetramethrin, either as the racemic mixture or the 1R, cis/trans isomer, is virtually non-irritating to the rabbit eye and is non-irritating to rabbit skin. In addition, neither the racemic mixture nor the 1R, cis/trans isomer is a sensitizer in guinea-pigs.

Tetramethrin is a type I pyrethroid. In mammals, tremor (T-syndrome) is the characteristic poisoning symptom.

When rats were fed tetramethrin at dietary levels of up to 5000 mg/kg diet for 91 days, reduced body weight gain was observed at 5000 mg/kg diet. The results from 3- or 6-month feeding studies using the 1R, cis/trans isomer in rats at dietary levels ranging from 25 mg/kg diet to 3000 mg/kg diet indicated that the no-observed-effect level was 200 mg/kg diet for males and 300 mg/kg diet for females (observations included decreases in the body weight gain and in final body weight, and effects on the kidney and liver). The effects on the liver were thought to be an adaptive response to the feeding of the corn oil vehicle.

The no-observed-effect level in a 26-week study in dogs was 1250 mg/kg diet.

When mice and rats were exposed to aerosolized tetramethrin by inhalation at a concentration of 200 mg/m^3 for 3-4 h/day for up to 4 weeks, no significant compound-related changes were observed. An additional inhalation study, in which rats were exposed to a mist (1.2-1.5 μm diameter droplets) of 1R,cis/trans isomer in deodorized kerosene at concentrations up to 87 mg/m^3, 3 h/day, 7 days/week for 28 days, indicated a no-observed-effect level of 49 mg/m^3. Toxic signs were noted only during the exposure period.

Neither tetramethrin nor its 1R,cis/trans isomers were mutagenic in a variety of *in vivo* and *in vitro* test systems, which investigated gene mutations, DNA damage, DNA repair, and chromosomal effects.

Three 104-week chronic/oncogenicity feeding studies have been conducted on tetramethrin, two in rats and one in mice. In mice, tetramethrin was fed at dose levels up to 1500 mg/kg diet. No oncogenic effects were observed. Decreased pituitary and thyroid/parathyroid weights were observed at 60 mg/kg diet or more. The no-observed-effect level for systemic effects was 12 mg/kg diet in mice. In the rat studies, the test animals were exposed to tetramethrin at dose levels up to 5000 mg/kg diet *in utero* and through long-term feeding. In both studies in rats, body weight gains were significantly lower in animals exposed to 3000 mg/kg diet or more. In addition, increases in liver weight were observed at these dose levels. The no-observed-effect level for systemic effects in both studies in rats was 1000 mg/kg diet. The incidence of testicular interstitial cell tumours at 3000 mg/kg diet or more was higher than the level in the concurrent control group in both studies. Testicular interstitial cell tumours occur spontaneously in aged rats, and the incidence can very greatly in control groups. This tumour is thought to be hormonally mediated. There was no evidence of malignancy and no evidence of this type of tumour in mice. It can be concluded that the tumorigenic effect, if real, is most unlikely to be relevant to human exposure.

Tetramethrin was not teratogenic or embryotoxic at dose levels up to 1000 mg/kg body weight in rats and up to 500 mg/kg body weight in rabbits (these were the highest dose levels tested). In a fertility study in which rats were given tetramethrin at dose levels up to 1000 mg/kg body weight per day, the no-observed-effect level for the parents' reproductive ability and growth of the fetuses was 300 mg/kg body weight per day. In a perinatal and post-natal reproduction study in rats, the no-observed-effect level was 100 mg/kg body weight per day (the highest level tested).

When dose levels of 1000-6000 mg/kg diet were tested in a one-generation reproduction study on tetramethrin in rats, the no-observed-effect level was 1000 mg/kg diet. Levels of the 1R,cis/trans isomer of 100-3000 mg/kg were tested in a two-generation reproduction study, which gave a no-observed-effect level of 500 mg/kg diet.

1.1.8 *Effects on human beings*

Although tetramethrin and its 1R isomer have been used for many years, there have been no reports of poisoning or adverse effects in human beings.

There are no indications that tetramethrin or its 1R-isomer will have an adverse effect on human beings if it continues to be used in low concentrations and only to control household pests.

1.2 Conclusions

(a) *General Population*: The exposure of the general population to tetramethrin, as it is currently used, is expected to be low. It is not likely to present a hazard if used as recommended.

(b) *Occupational Exposure*: When good work practices, hygiene measures and safety precautions are followed, tetramethrin is unlikely to present a hazard to those occupationally exposed.

(c) *Environment*: It is highly unlikely that tetramethrin or its degradation products will reach levels that could cause adverse environmental effects.

1.3 Recommendations

Although tetramethrin and its 1R isomer have been used for many years with no reports of adverse effects in humans, observations of human exposure should continue.

2. IDENTITY, PHYSICAL AND CHEMICAL PROPERTIES, ANALYTICAL METHODS

2.1 Identity

Molecular formula: $C_{19}H_{25}NO_4$

Chemical structure:

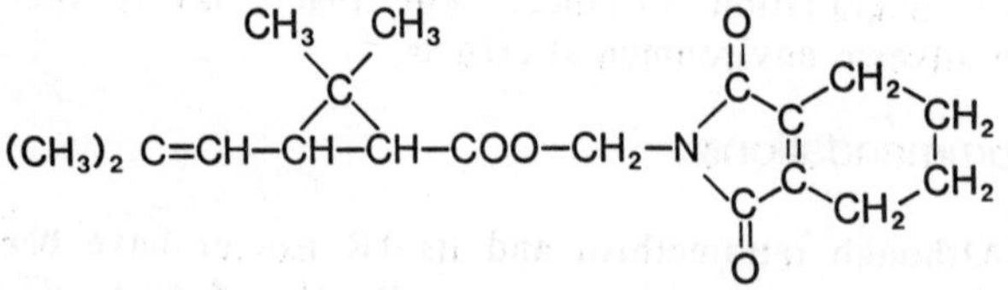

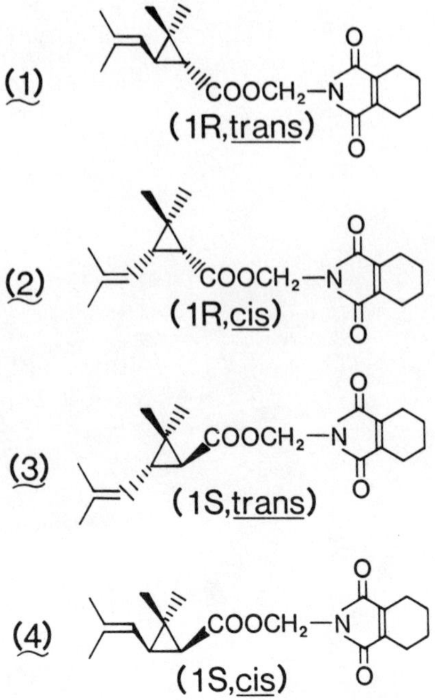

(1) (1R,*trans*)

(2) (1R,*cis*)

(3) (1S,*trans*)

(4) (1S,*cis*)

Fig. 1. Chemical structures of four stereoisomers.

Tetramethrin was first synthesized in 1964 by Kato et al. [19] and is prepared by the esterificaton of (1RS,*cis,trans*)-2,2-dimethyl-3-(2,2-dimethylvinyl)-cyclopropanecarboxylic acid (chrysanthemic acid) with 3,4,5,6-tetrahydrophthalimidomethyl alcohol. It is a mixture of four stereoisomers (Fig. 1). The cis:trans ratio is reported to be 1:4 and the optical ratio of 1R:1S is 1:1 (racemic). Thus its composition is roughly 4:1:4:1 for the [IR,trans], [IR,cis], [IS,trans], and [IS,cis] isomers. The [1R,trans] isomer is the most active biologically of the isomers, followed by the [1R,cis] isomer. Neo-Pynamin Forte is a mixture of the [1R,cis,] and [IR,trans] isomers in the ratio of 1:4 (Table 1).

2.2 Physical and Chemical Properties

Some physical and chemical properties of tetramethrin are given in Table 2.

No data are available for boiling point and *n*-octanol/water partition coefficient. Technical grade tetramethrin is stable to heat (50 °C for 6 months) but unstable to light and air and to alkaline condition [30, 31, 76].

2.3 Analytical Methods

Dislodgeable residues of tetramethrin can be analysed by dual-wavelength densitometry after clean-up of the hexane washings by high-performance silica gel thin-layer chromatography (Table 3). To analyse technical grade tetramethrin, the product and tributoxyethyl phosphate (an internal standard) were dissolved in acetone, and the solution was injected into a gas chromatograph equipped with flame ionization detector (FID) [37]). Analysis of tetramethrin formulations can also be carried out using high performance liquid chromatography (HPLC) with an infra-red selective detector [42].

Table 1. Chemical identity of tetramethrins of various stereoisomeric compositions

Common name/ CAS Registry no./ NIOSH Accession no.[a]	CAS Index name (9CI) Stereospecific name[b,c]	Stereoisomeric composition[d]	Synonyms and trade names
Tetramethrin[e] (racemic mixture) 7696-12-0 GZ173000[a]	Cyclopropanecarboxylic acid, 2,2-dimethyl-3-(2-methyl-1-propenyl)-, (1,3,4,5,6,7-hexahydro-1,3-dioxo-2*H*-isoindol-2-yl)methyl ester	(1):(2):(3):(4) = 4:1:4:1	Tetramethrine, Phthalthrin, Neo-Pynamin, FMC-9260
	3,4,5,6-Tetrahydrophthalimidomethyl (1RS,*cis,trans*)-2,2-dimethyl-3-(2,2-dimethylvinyl)cyclopropane-carboxylate or 3,4,5,6-Tetrahydrophthalimidomethyl-(1RS,*cis,trans*)-chrysanthemate		
(+)-*trans*-Tetramethrin	Same as tetramethrin		(+)-*trans*-Phthalthrin
GZ1710000[a]	3,4,5,6-Tetrahydrophthalimidomethyl (1R,*trans*)-chrysanthemate		
(+)-Tetramethrin	Same as tetramethrin	(1):(2) = 4:1	Neo-Pynamin Forte
GZ1720000[a]	3,4,5,6-Tetrahydrophthalimidomethyl (1R,*cis,trans*)-chrysanthemate		

a Registry of Toxic Effects of Chemical Substances (RTECS) (1981-82 edition).
b (1R), d, (+) or (1S), l, (-) in the acid part of tetramethrin signify the same stereospecific conformation, respectively.
c Chrysanthemic acid is a name of the acid that forms the acid part.
d Numbers in parentheses identify the structures shown in Fig. 1.
e ISO common name: common names for pesticides and other agrochemicals approved by the Technical Committee of the International Organization for Standardization.

Table 2. Some physical and chemical properties of tetramethrin

	Racemic mixture	(1R) isomer
Physical state	crystalline solid	viscous liquid
Colour	colourless	yellow or brown
Odour	pyrethrum-like	pyrethrum-like
Relative molecular mass	331.45	331.45
Melting point (°C)	60 - 80	
Water solubility	4.6 mg/litre (30 °C)	2 - 4 mg/litre (23 °C)
Solubility in organic solvents	soluble[a]	soluble[b]
Density	d_{20}^{20} 1.108 (20 °C)	d_{25}^{25} 1.11
Vapour pressure (20 °C)	4.67×10^{-3} mPa (3.5×10^{-8} mmHg)	3.2×10^{-4} mPa (2.4×10^{-9} mmHg)
(30 °C)	9.46×10^{-1} mPa (7.1×10^{-6} mmHg)	

a Methanol (53 g/kg), hexane (20 g/kg), xylene (1 kg/kg), acetone, toluene.
b Hexane (>1 kg/kg), methanol, xylene.

Table 3. Analytical methods for tetramethrin

Sample	Sample preparation				Determination	% Recovery	Reference
	Extraction Solvent	Partition	Clean up: Column	Clean up: Elution	Detection method and conditions	(fortification level)[a]	
Environmental analysis							
Dish[b] Apple Spinach (dislodgeable residue)	*n*-hexane	*n*-hexane/ CH_3CN	HPTLC	benzene/CCl_4(1/1) *n*-hexane/ether/ formic acid (70/30/1) Rf = 0.35	dual-wavelength densitometry R = 370 nm; S = 230 nm	76-95 (0.3 mg) 88 (0.3 mg) 94 (0.3 mg)	61
Product analysis							
Technical grade	acetone				FID-GC, N_2 40 ml/min, 1-m column, 2% DEGS, 200°C, 12.4 min (retention time)		37
Formulations					HPLC, 0.01-mm Partisil column, $CC1_4$: CH_2Cl_2: $CHCl_3$: CH_3CN = 42.5: 42.5: 14.85: 0.15, with IR detection		42

a fortification level = concentration of tetramethrin added to control samples for the measurements of recovery.
b Wood, glass, china, or polypropylene.

3. SOURCES AND LEVELS OF HUMAN AND ENVIRONMENTAL EXPOSURE

3.1 Industrial Production

Tetramethrin was first marketed in 1964 [15]. Although no information on production volume is publicly available, it is estimated that a few hundred tonnes are manufactured annually in the world, mainly in Japan.

3.2 Use Patterns

Tetramethrin is used in aerosol formulations, emulsifiable concentrates, and mosquito coils for indoor pest control. It is also formulated in combination with other insecticides (e.g., resmethrin) and synergists (e.g., piperonyl butoxide).

3.3 Residues in Food

Tetramethrin is not used on food crops.

3.4 Exposure Levels from Household Use

With conventional household aerosol spraying or mosquito coil fumigation, the aerial levels of tetramethrin and its 1R isomer are unlikely to exceed 0.5 mg/m^3 [38].

3.5 Environmental Levels

No data are available.

4. ENVIRONMENTAL TRANSPORT, DISTRIBUTION, AND TRANSFORMATION

4.1 Abiotic Degradation in Air and Water

The photodegradation pathways for tetramethrin are summarized in Fig. 2. Exposure of *trans*-[carboxyl-^{14}C] tetramethrin (5)[a], as a thin film (0.1-0.3 mg/cm^2), to sunlight resulted in rapid degradation. During a 2-h exposure (30% conversion), the major photoproducts were the (1RS)-epoxides (7) (14% of the reaction mixture), the aldehyde derivative (10) (19%) oxidized at the (E)-methyl group in the acid moiety, the caronaldehyde derivative (16) (6%) from cleavage upon ozonolysis, and the allylic hydroperoxide (15) (6%) from the hydroperoxidation at the 1′-position of the isobutenyl moiety. In addition, small amounts of *cis*-tetramethrin (14) (2%), the alcohol (9) (5%) and carboxy (11) (3%) derivatives oxidized at the (E)-methyl group, and the hydroxy derivative (6) (3%) at the allylic methylene group in the alcohol moiety and its epoxide (8) (2%) were detected. These identified ester photoproducts accounted for approximately 80% in a 5% conversion but only approximately 20% in a 50-70% conversion. Chrysanthemic acid (12) and *N*-(hydroxymethyl)-tetrahydrophthalimide (13), formed by ester bond cleavage, were minor products, and much of the radiocarbon remained at the origin on the TLC plate. The *cis/trans* isomerization was an inefficient reaction in an oxygen-containing atmosphere [50].

[a] Numbers in parentheses refer to numbered chemical structures in Figures 2 and 3.

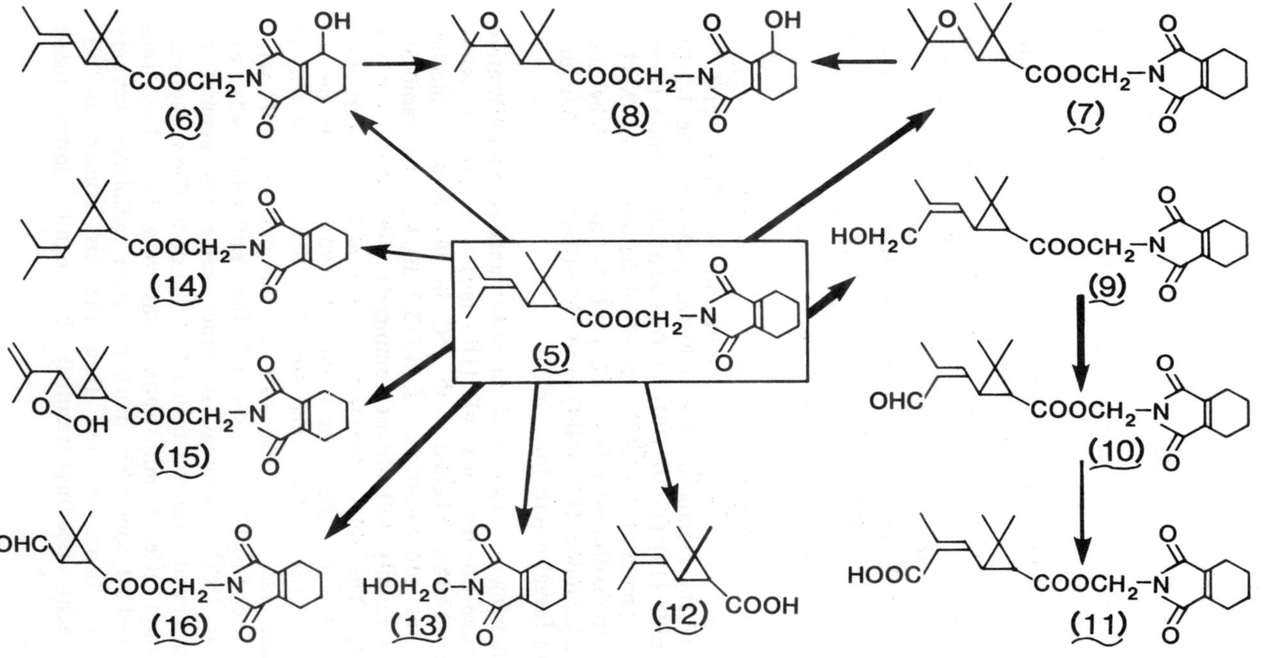

Fig. 2. Photodegradation pathways of tetramethrin.

5. KINETICS AND METABOLISM

5.1 Metabolism in Mammals

The metabolic pathways of tetramethrin in mammals are summarized in Fig. 3.

Tetramethrin is readily absorbed and excreted by rats. Following a single oral administration of [1RS,*trans*]-tetramethrin (17], labelled with ^{14}C at the carbonyl group of the alcohol moiety, to male Wistar rats at a concentration of 500 mg/kg, 47% and 42% of the radiolabel were excreted into the urine and faeces, respectively, during the subsequent 2 days and 95% was recovered during the 5-day period that followed dosing. The tissue levels during the first 2 days after administration were very low and the tetramethrin content in tissues was less than 0.01% of the dosed radioactivity. Unmetabolized *trans*-tetramethrin (17) was not excreted into the urine, and the major urinary metabolite was 3-hydroxy-cyclohexane-1,2-dicarboximide (19) (3-OH-HPI) in free and glucuronide forms. *N*-(Hydroxymethyl)-3,4,5,6-tetrahydrophthalimide (20) (MTI), 3,4,5,6-tetrahydrophthalimide (21) (TPI), and cyclohexane-1,2-dicarboximide (22) (HPI) were identified as minor urinary and faecal metabolites [36].

Following a single oral or subcutaneous administration to Sprague-Dawley rats of [1R,*trans*]- or [1R,*cis*]-tetramethrin (17,18), labelled with ^{14}C in the acid or alcohol moieties at concentrations of 3.2-5.3 mg/kg, the radiocarbon was rapidly and almost completely eliminated from the rat body. The total recoveries 7 days after administration were 93-97% for the trans isomer and 90-101% for the cis isomer (approximately equal amounts being eliminated in urine and faeces). In the case of the oral dose of acid-labelled tetramethrin, 1-3% of the radiolabel was excreted as $^{14}CO_2$, whereas in other cases the amount of $^{14}CO_2$ accounted for less than 1% of the dose. The tissue residue 7 days after administration was very low. The trans isomer yielded somewhat more complete radiolabel recovery and lower tissue residues than the cis isomer. In addition, acid labelling resulted in slightly lower tissue

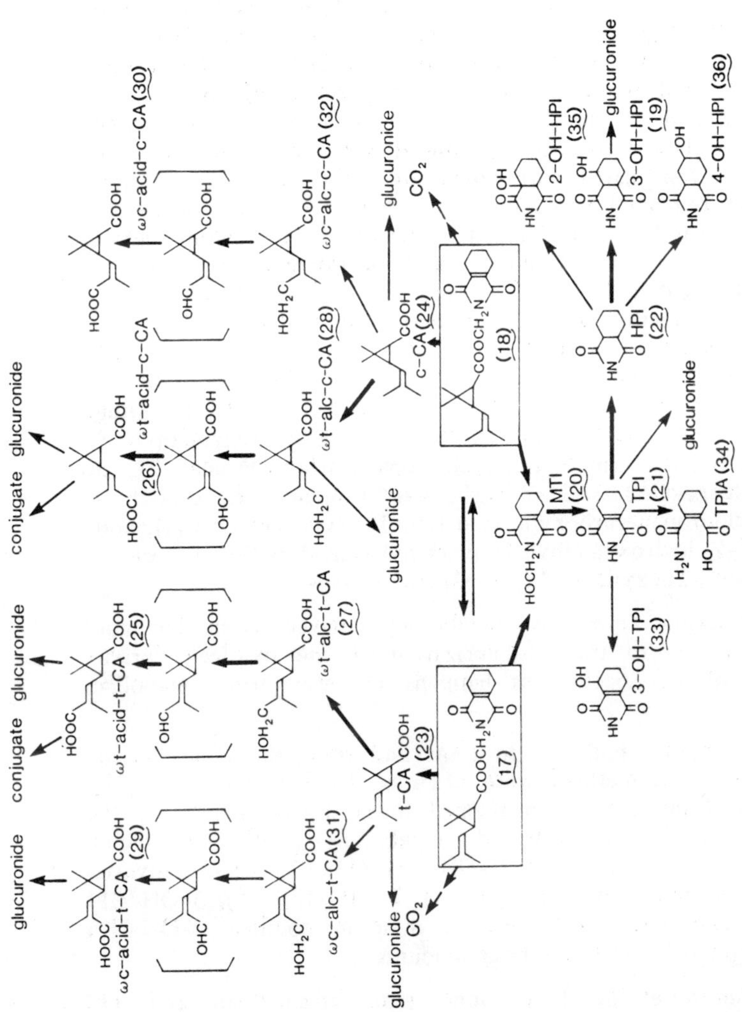

Fig. 3. Metabolic pathways of tetramethrin in mammals.

residues than did alcohol labelling. However, there were no significant differences, according to sex or administration route, in the total radiocarbon recoveries and tissue residue levels [18]. The major metabolic reactions of both [1R,*trans*]- and [1R,*cis*]-tetramethrin were ester cleavage, loss of the hydroxymethyl group from the alcohol moiety, reduction of the 1-2 bond of the alcohol moiety, and oxidation at the isobutenyl group of the acid moiety and at the 2-, 3-, and 4-positions of the alcohol moiety. The metabolites produced via these reactions were in part conjugated with glucuronic acid. None of the trans isomer remained unmetabolized, whereas 0.3-1.2% of the cis isomer was found unchanged in the faeces. The major metabolites from the acid moiety of both isomers were chrysanthemic acid (23, 24) (CA) and its derivatives oxidized at the trans-methyl of the isobutenyl group. 3-(2′-E-Carboxy-1′-propenyl)-2,2-dimethyl-1-cyclopropanecarboxylic acid (25, 26) (*ωt*-acid-*t,c*-CA) accounted for 17-27% and 7-9% of the dose of the trans and cis isomers, respectively. Other significant metabolites were 3-(2′-E-hydroxymethyl-1′-propenyl)-2,2-dimethyl-1-cyclopropanecarboxylic acid (27, 28) (*ωt*-alc-*t,c*-CA), 3-(2′-Z-carboxy-1′-propenyl)-2,2-dimethyl-1-cyclopropanecarboxylic acid (29, 30) (*ωc*-acid-*t,c*-CA), and 3-(2′-Z-hydroxymethyl-1′-propenyl)-2,2-dimethyl-1-cyclopropanecarboxylic acid (31, 32) (*ωc*-alc-*t,c*-CA).

Judging from the metabolites derived from the acid moiety, cis to trans isomerization of the oxidized derivatives of CA occurs, as happens in resmethrin metabolism [60].

Although both cis to trans and trans to cis isomerizations of tetramethrin were observed by Kaneko et al. [18], cis to trans conversion seemed to be predominant. On the other hand, the detected metabolites from the alcohol moiety were TPI, HPI, 3-OH-TPI (33), 3,4,5,6-tetrahydrophthalic acid amide (34) (TPIA), 2-OH-HPI (35), 3-OH-HPI (19), and 4-OH-HPI (36). Of these metabolites, 2-OH-HPI was found in relatively large amounts.

Smith et al. [55] found that tetramethrin and TPI readily underwent the Michael addition with thiols. The tetramethrin-gluthathione (GSH) conjugate was formed under physiological conditions in the presence of mouse liver homogenate fractions, probably by a non-enzymatic reaction. The soluble thiol level of mouse liver was decreased by intraperitoneal administration of TPI. However, mercapturic acid and GSH conjugates of tetramethrin were not detected in the bile or urine of rats or mice treated intraperitoneally with tetramethrin.

5.2 Enzymatic Systems for Biotransformation

When alcohol- or acid-labelled [1RS,*trans*]-tetramethrin (1 mmol/litre) was incubated for 1 h at 37 °C with 30 mg protein of a rat liver subcellular fraction (i.e. nuclei plus mitochondria, microsomes, and soluble fraction), the microsomes and nuclei plus mitochondria fractions were active in degrading tetramethrin. Rat microsomal fraction degraded [1RS,*trans*]-tetramethrin to CA, MTI, and TPI in the absence of NADPH. In the presence of NADPH, tetramethrin was more rapidly degraded to yield oxidized tetramethrin (*wt*-alc-, *wt*-ald-, and *wt*-acid-tetramethrin), oxidized CA (*wt*-alc-, *wt*-ald-, and *wt*-acid-CA), TPI, and unidentified metabolites in larger amounts. The major metabolite TPI was shown to be produced non-enzymatically from MTI. The degradation rate of tetramethrin was greatly reduced by the inhibition of ester hydrolysis with paraoxon [57].

6. EFFECTS ON ORGANISMS IN THE ENVIRONMENT

As the use of tetramethrin is limited to indoor pest control, there is a paucity of data concerning its effect on the environment.

6.1 Aquatic Organisms

Data on the toxicity of tetramethrin to non-target aquatic organisms are given in Table 4.

Tetramethrin is highly acutely toxic to fish in laboratory tests, the 96-h LC_{50}s for two species being approximately 20 µg/litre[a]. The 48-h LC_{50} for killifish is about 200 µg/litre, with a no-observed-effect level (NOEL) of 50 µg/litre [33]. The NOEL for *Daphnia pulex* was reported by Miyamoto [33] to be 50 µg/litre for racemic tetramethrin and 10 µg/litre for [1R,*trans*]- or [1R,*cis*]-tetramethrin.

6.2 Terrestrial Organisms

Tetramethrin has low toxicity to birds. The acute oral LD_{50} for Bobwhite quail is >2510 mg/kg body weight, and the 8-day dietary LC_{50} to Mallard duck and Bobwhite quail is >5620 mg/kg[a].

Tetramethrin is toxic to bees [14].

[a] Written comment from US EPA to IPCS, 1987.

Table 4. Acute toxicity of tetramethrin to non-target aquatic organisms

Species	Size	Parameter	Toxicity (mg/litre)	Formulation	System	Temperature (°C)	Reference
Fish							
Killifish	adult	48-h LC_{50}	0.2	Technical	Static	25	33
(*Oryzias latipes*)	adult	48-h LC_{50}	0.2	(+)-trans	Static	25	33
	adult	48-h LC_{50}	0.15	(+)-cis	Static	25	33
Bluegill sunfish (*Lepomis macrochirur*)		96-h LC_{50}	0.019				*a*
Rainbow trout (*Salmo gairdneri*)		96-h LC_{50}	0.021				*a*
Arthropods							
Daphnia pulex		3-h LC_{50}	>50	Technical	Static	25	33
		3-h LC_{50}	>50	(+)-trans	Static	25	33
		3-h LC_{50}	>50	(+)-cis	Static	25	33

a Written comment from US EPA to IPCS, 1987.

7. EFFECTS ON EXPERIMENTAL ANIMALS AND *IN VITRO* TEST SYSTEMS

7.1 Single Exposures

The acute toxicity of tetramethrin to rats and mice is low (Table 5).

Table 5. Acute toxicity of tetramethrin to rats and mice

Compound	Species	Sex	Route	LD_{50} (mg/kg body weight)	Reference
Racemic	rat	M,F	oral	4600	41
	rat[a]	M,F	oral[b]	> 5000	17
	rat	M,F	dermal[b]	> 10 000	41
	mouse[a]	M	oral[b]	1920	17
	mouse[a]	F	oral[b]	2000	17
(1R,*cis/trans*)-	rat[a]	M,F	oral[b]	> 5000	16
	rat	M,F	subcutaneous	> 5000	16
	rat	M	intraperitoneal	770	16
	rat	F	intraperitoneal	548	16
	rat	M,F	dermal(>24 h)[b]	> 5000	16
	mouse[a]	M	oral	1060	16
	mouse[a]	F	oral	1040	16
	mouse	M	subcutaneous	2020	16
	mouse	F	subcutaneous	1950	16
	mouse	M	intraperitoneal	631	16
	mouse	F	intraperitoneal	527	16
	mouse	M,F	dermal (>24 h)[b]	> 5000	16
	rabbit		dermal (>24 h)[b]	> 2000	20

[a] Animals were not fasted.
[b] Corn oil was used as vehicle.

Sprague-Dawley rats (10 of each sex per group) were exposed to a respirable mist (droplet diameter of 1.2-1.5 μm) of [1R,*cis/trans*]-tetramethrin (technical grade, 95.6% purity) in deodorized kerosene (0, 26, 131, 243, 595, and 1180 mg active ingredient per m^3 air) for a duration of 3 h. At 131 mg/m^3 or more, salivation, hyper-excitability, irregular respiration, urinary incontinence, muscular fibrillation, limb paralysis, decrease in spontaneous activity, and other toxic signs were observed in males and females. At 1180 mg/m^3, 10% of female animals died, but the body weight gain was similar to that of the control rats. The no-observed-effect level (NOEL) for inhalation of the compound in rats was 26 mg/m^3, and the LC_{50} value was >1180 mg/m^3 in both sexes [58].

The toxic symptoms observed following [1R,*cis/trans*]-tetramethrin administration were hyperexcitability, muscle twitching, tremor, ataxia, irregular respiration, and depression. Mice were invariably more susceptible than rats. No differences in susceptibility were observed between male and female animals [16, 17, 33].

7.2 Irritation and Sensitization

7.2.1 *Eye irritation*

In a study by Okuno et al. [39], 50 mg of the technical product (91.3% purity) was instilled in one eye of Japanese albino male rabbits. The treated eye was washed with distilled water 5 min (group I) or 24 h (group II) thereafter. The conjunctiva, cornea, and pupil were examined, 1, 24, 72 h and 7, 14, and 21 days after application. No particular changes were noted except that a very slight erythema and oedema of the conjunctiva was transiently observed in the rabbits in group II.

In a separate study, 0.1 ml [1R,*cis/trans*]-tetramethrin (technical grade, 95.6% purity) was applied to one eye of Japanese albino rabbits. The treated eye was subsequently washed in five rabbits but not in three other rabbits. The material did not produce any lesions in the cornea or iris of the treated eyes that were not washed, but slight hyperemia and/or chemosis of the conjunctiva was observed 1 h after application. In the washed eyes, slight hyperemia of the conjunctiva was observed in all animals 1 h after treatment. These changes, however, had disappeared by 48 h after application in the unwashed eyes and 24 h in the washed eyes. The irritating potency of the material was judged to be minimal in the unwashed eyes and negative in the washed eyes [11].

7.2.2 *Skin irritation*

In a study by Okuno et al. [39], 0.5 g of the technical product (91.3% purity) was applied on a lint patch (3.8 x 3.8 cm) to the abraded or intact skin of six rabbits. The skin was assessed for severity of erythema and oedema 4, 24, 48, 72 h and 7, 14, and 21 days after application, but no particular changes were noted.

When 0.5 ml [1R,*cis/trans*]-tetramethrin (technical grade, 95.6% purity) was applied on a lint patch (2.5 x 2.5 cm) to abraded or intact skin on the back of rabbits, again no irritating reactions such as erythema and oedema were observed [11].

7.2.3 *Sensitization*

In a skin-sensitization study of tetramethrin in guinea-pigs, Hartley male guinea-pigs (seven per group) were sensitized ten times at intervals of one or two days by intracutaneous injections (first injection: 0.05 ml, subsequent ones: 0.1 ml) of a 1% solution of the technical product (91.3% purity) in corn oil. The sensitized animals were then challenged against the same concentration in the same manner (0.5 ml injection) 14 days later, but no skin-sensitization reaction was noted [40].

In another skin-sensitization test on Hartley male guinea-pigs, 0.5 ml [1R,*cis/trans*]-tetramethrin (technical product, 95.6% purity) in 0.5 ml acetone was applied topically by lint patch to the back of animals ten times (three times per week). The animals were challenged in the same manner 2 weeks after the last sensitizing treatment, but no allergic reactions were observed 24 h later [12].

7.3 Short-Term Exposure Studies

7.3.1 *Oral*

When groups of 10 male Wistar rats were maintained for 91 days on a diet containing 0, 500, 1000, 3000, or 5000 mg tetramethrin/kg diet, there was a reduced rate of body weight gain at 5000 mg/kg but not at 3000 mg/kg or less. The liver glycogen level was reduced at 3000 mg/kg and 5000 mg/kg. The kidney, spleen, heart, small intestine, and brain showed no abnormal signs, either macroscopically or microscopically, and there were no significant changes in blood parameters. There was no increase in the protein or glucose levels in the urine of test animals [59].

When technical (1R,*cis*/*trans*)-tetramethrin in corn oil was administered to Sprague-Dawley rats for 3 or 6 months at 0, 100, 300, 1000, or 3000 mg/kg diet, no treatment-related changes were observed in clinical signs, or food and water consumption, or in an ophthalmological examination. However, the body weight gain and final body weight of males and females in the 3000-mg/kg group were significantly lower than those of the controls. There were slight increases in urine protein level in the rats fed more than 1000 mg/kg and in serum calcium level in the male rats fed more than 300 mg/kg. During a histopathological examination, eosinophilic bodies in tubular epithelial cells and hyaline droplets in kidney tubular epithelium cytoplasm were observed in males fed 3000 mg/kg diet, along with an increase in relative organ weight. There were dose-dependent increases in absolute and relative liver weight in all treated male rats and in female rats fed more than 1000 mg/kg diet. There were also slightly higher serum cholesterol concentrations in rats of both sexes fed more than 1000 mg/kg and a significant reduction in liver lipid content among males fed 1000 mg/kg or more. However, these liver effects were not accompanied by damage to hepatocytes and were therefore considered to be an adaptation to the corn oil without toxicological significance. Furthermore, there were no marked effects, even at 200 mg/kg, when an additional subchronic study was conducted at tetramethrin levels of 25, 50, 100, and 200 mg/kg diet without corn oil in order to confirm the NOEL in male rats. The NOEL for tetramethrin in rats in the 6-month study was concluded to be 200 mg/kg diet for males and 300 mg/kg diet for females [16].

When technical grade tetramethrin (94.6% purity) was administered for 26 weeks to beagle dogs (six of each sex per group) at levels of 0, 1250, 2500, and 5000 mg/kg diet, nervousness and tremors were observed in both males and females at 2500 and 5000 mg/kg diet. A lack of oestrus activity in females was also noted clinically and a lack of corpora lutea was confirmed histologically at 5000 mg/kg diet. Absolute liver weight was increased in males at 2500 and 5000 mg/kg and relative liver weight was significantly increased in males and females at 5000 mg/kg. Decreased absolute/relative ovary weights were noted for females at 5000 mg/kg. No other treatment-related changes were observed with respect to survival, body weight gain, food consumption, haematology, urinalysis, ophthalmology, gross pathology or histopathology. The NOEL was 1250 mg/kg diet [43].

In a study by Weir & Crus (1966), groups of three male and three female beagle dogs were fed tetramethrin dissolved in corn oil for 13 weeks at levels of 0, 1250, 2500, and 5000 mg/kg diet. There were no effects on haematological, clinical chemistry, or urinary parameters. Organ weights were not affected by the treatment, and there were no significant histopathological findings. Clinical signs were not recorded. The NOEL was >5000 mg/kg diet.

7.3.2 *Inhalation*

Sprague-Dawley rats (10 of each sex per group) were exposed to a respirable mist (droplet diameter of 1-2 μm) of tetramethrin at concentrations of 0, 26, 49, and 87 mg active ingredient per m^3 air, 3 h a day, 7 days a week, for a period of 28 days. At 87 mg/m^3, irregular respiration, slight salivation, and hyperexcitability were observed as toxic signs every day during the exposure period, but no cumulative toxicity was noted. There were no compound-related effects on body weight gain, food and water consumption, urinalysis, haematology, biochemistry, organ weight, and histopathology. The NOEL in subacute inhalation was considered to be 49 mg/m^3 [58]. This NOEL is approximately 100 times higher than the aerial concentration attained during normal use of tetramethrin [33].

7.4 Long-Term Exposures and Carcinogenicity

Appraisal

Testicular interstitial cell tumours occur spontaneously in aged rats, and the incidence can vary greatly in control groups. This tumour is believed to be hormonally mediated. There was no evidence of malignancy in three rat studies and no evidence of this type of tumour in mice. It can be concluded that the tumorigenic effect, if real, is most unlikely to be relevant to human exposure.

When tetramethrin (technical grade) was administered to Sprague-Dawley CRCDR rats (50 of each sex per group, F_{1A} weanlings from parental animals pre-treated with the compound at dose levels of 1000, 3000, and 6000 mg/kg diet) at dose levels of 0, 1000, 3000, or 5000 mg/kg diet for 104 weeks, no compound-related effects were detected in investigations of appearance, behaviour, survival, haematology, blood chemistry, urinalysis, eye examination, and organ weight at up to 5000 mg/kg diet. However, the body weight gain of male and female rats fed 3000 mg/kg or more was significantly lower than that of controls. The incidence for testicular interstitial cell tumours was increased at dose levels of 3000 mg/kg or more [49].

Tetramethrin (technical grade, 90.0/93.6% purity) was tested for long-term toxic effects and tumorigenic potential in Sprague-Dawley CRCDR and Long-Evans hooded rats by *in utero* exposure and 104-week chronic exposure at dose levels of 0, 200, 1000, and 5000 mg/kg diet. No distinct compound-related effects were observed in either strain with regard to fertility rate, mortality, clinical signs, and clinical laboratory data. However, body weight gains were significantly lower in both strains at 5000 mg/kg diet, and absolute and relative liver weights were increased in both strains at 5000 mg/kg diet. The incidence of interstitial cell tumours in both strains at 5000 mg/kg diet was above the level in the concurrent control groups [44].

When tetramethrin (technical product, 93.3% purity) was fed daily to $B6C3F_1$ mice (dose levels of 0, 12, 60, 300, or 1500 mg/kg diet) for 104 weeks, there were no significant dose-related changes in survival, clinical signs, mean body weight, or food consumption. However, the mortality of male mice at 300 mg/kg was significantly lower than that of control males. The absolute and relative weight of pituitary and thyroid/parathyroid glands was decreased for males fed 60 mg/kg diet or more. Absolute spleen weights were also decreased for males fed 300 mg/kg diet or more. However, gross and microscopic examination of these tissues did not reveal any treatment-related histomorphological changes. There were no other histopathological findings attributable to tetramethrin administration. The NOEL was considered to be 12 mg/kg diet [45].

7.5 Mutagenicity

The results of mutagenicity tests on tetramethrin are summarized in Table 6.

Ding et al. [2] reported the induction of unscheduled DNA synthesis in human amnion FL cells by tetramethrin (72% industrial grade of unknown origin). The same product gave weakly positive results in an Ames test with Salmonella typhimurium TA 97. It is not clear if the effect was caused by tetramethrin itself or by the unidentified (28%) portion of the industrial grade material.

7.6 Reproduction, Embryotoxicity, and Teratogenicity

In a study by Miyamoto [33], groups of 10-15 pregnant New Zealand white rabbits received tetramethrin orally on days 6-18 of gestation at doses of 0, 30, or 90 mg/kg per day. Fetuses were obtained by caesarean section prior to parturition and were examined for external and skeletal abnormalities. Seven extra pregnant animals were allowed to give birth naturally and the pups were examined for several weeks to check their growth and development. No significant adverse effects were observed.

Tetramethrin (technical product) was orally administered (dose levels of 0, 100, 300, and 1000 mg/kg body weight per day) to 6-week-old male Slc: SD rats (SPF, 20 per group) for not less than 9 weeks and to 9-week-old females (20 per group) for 2 weeks of the non-pregnant period and up to day 7 of pregnancy. The effects of the material on the mating ability of male and female animals and on the fetuses were investigated. In males, the liver weight increased at all dose levels and a kidney weight increase was noted at 1000 mg/kg. Salivation and a slower body weight increase were observed during the latter half of the administration period at 300 and 1000 mg/kg. However, no effects on the reproductive ability of males were noted. In females, no changes were observed in the rate of pregnancy, but there were effects on the sexual cycle and

Table 6. Mutagenicity studies on tetramethrin

Test System	Test object	Concentration	Purity/ Compound	Results	Reference
Ames test	S. typhimurium TA 1535 TA 1538	up to 10 mg/plate without activation	93 - 100%	Negative	33
Ames test	*Escherichia coli* W 3623 W 3012	up to 10 mg/plate without activation	93 - 100%	Negative	33
Ames test	S. typhimurium TA 100 TA 98 TA 1535 TA 1538	1 - 10 000 µg/plate with and without activation	technical racemic	Negative	56
Ames test	S. typhimurium TA 100 TA 98 TA 1535 TA 1537 TA 97	100 - 5000 µg/plate with and without activation	94.0% racemic	Negative	81
Ames test	*E. coli* WP2 *uvr* A	100 - 5000 µg/plate with and without activation	94.0% racemic	Negative	81

Table 6 (contd).

Test System	Test object	Concentration	Purity/ Compound	Results	Reference
Ames test	S. typhimurium TA 100 TA 98 TA 1535 TA 1537 TA 1538	10 - 5000 µg/plate with and without activation	95.6%, 1R,*cis/trans*	Negative	22
Ames test	*E. coli* WP2 *uvr* A	10 - 5000 µg/plate	95.6%, 1R,*cis/trans*	Negative	22
Ames test	S. typhimurium TA 97	5 - 500 µg/plate without activation	72% industrial grade	Positive[a]	2
Rec-assay	*Bacillus subtilis* M45 *rec*⁻ and H17 (wild type)	1 - 10 000 µg/disk	technical racemic	Negative	56
Rec-assay	*Bacillus subtilis* M45 *rec*⁻ and H17 (wild type)	50 - 5000 µg/disk	95.6%, 1R,*cis/trans*	Negative	22
Host-mediated assay	ICR male mice S. typhimurium G46	200 - 1000 mg/kg body weight (oral)	technical racemic	Negative	56

Table 6 (contd).

In vivo chromosomal aberration	ICR male mice bone marrow	1200, 2400, 5000 mg/kg body weight (ip)	93.4% racemic	Negative	80
In vivo chromosomal aberration	ICR male mice bone marrow	150, 300, 600 mg/kg body weight (ip)	95.6%, 1R,*cis/trans*	Negative	13
Unscheduled DNA synthesis	Human amnion FL cells	Not recorded	72%, industrial grade	Positive[a]	2
Unscheduled DNA synthesis	Rat hepatocyte primary cultures	0, 0.2, 1, 5, 25, 50, and 100 μg/ml	94.0% racemic	Negative	21

a The test material was of unknown origin and it was unclear whether or not positive results were due to the 28% impurities.

an ovulation-inhibiting effect at 1000 mg/kg. In fetuses, growth inhibition was suspected at 1000 mg/kg. However, all these changes were slight. The NOEL was considered to be 300 mg/kg body weight per day for reproductive ability of parents and growth of fetuses [51].

Tetramethrin (technical product) was orally administered (dose levels of 0, 100, 300, and 1000 mg/kg body weight per day) to Slc: SD rats (SPF, 30 per group) on days 7-17 of pregnancy, and its effects on the dams, fetuses, and growth of pups were investigated. In dams, an inhibition of body weight increase and a decrease of food consumption were observed at 1000 mg/kg, in addition to an increase in liver and kidney weights at the time of caesarean section. In fetuses, no abnormalities such as embryo lethality, growth inhibition, or teratogenic effects were detected. In addition, the tetramethrin had no effect on the growth of the young after birth or on the reproductive ability of the offspring. The NOEL was considered to be 300 mg/kg body weight per day for the dams and >1000 mg/kg body weight per day for teratogenicity [52].

When tetramethrin (technical product) was orally administered at dose levels of 0, 50, 150, or 500 mg/kg body weight per day to pregnant Japanese white rabbits, (10 per group) on days 8-18 of pregnancy, a slight transient decline in the body weight of the dams was noted in the middle of the treatment period at 500 mg/kg. No adverse effects such as embryo lethality, inhibition of fetal growth, or teratogenic action were observed at any dose level. The NOEL for teratogenicity in rabbits was considered to be >500 mg/kg body weight per day [53].

Tetramethrin (technical product) was orally administered (dose levels of 0, 100, 300, and 1000 mg/kg body weight per day) to Slc: SD rats (SPF, 20 per group) from day 17 of gestation to day 21 of lactation (perinatal and postnatal period). In dams, a liver weight increase was noted at 300 and 1000 mg/kg but there were no abnormalities at delivery or during lactation. Tetramethrin had no detectable effects on the survival rate of pups, growth and development, sensory function, motor function, learning ability, or reproductive ability. The NOEL was considered to be 100 mg/kg body weight per day for dams and >1000 mg/kg body weight per day for pups [54].

In studies by Rutter [48], tetramethrin (technical grade) was administered to Sprague-Dawley rats at dose levels of 0, 1000, 3000, and 6000 mg/kg diet for 9 weeks through weaning of the F_{1A} generation. Body weight reduction occurred at 6000 mg/kg diet in the parent rats. The lactation index was depressed for the F_{1A} generation at 6000 mg/kg diet, and the weaning body weights for both sexes of the F_{1A} generation were reduced at doses of 3000 mg/kg diet or more. There were no other compound-related adverse effects. The NOEL was considered to be 1000 mg/kg diet.

(1R,*cis/trans*)-tetramethrin (technical product, 93.4% purity) was administered at dose levels of 0, 100, 500, and 3000 mg/kg diet to two successive generations of Sprague-Dawley CDR albino rats to determine the effects on the growth and reproductive performance. The body weights of parental females were significantly lower during the pre-mating growth, gestation, lactation, and post-weaning periods, and the body weight of offsprings of both generations decreased during lactation at 3000 mg/kg diet. Slight bile duct hyperplasia was noted in F_1 females sacrificed after a 30-day feeding period following weaning of the F_2 offspring at 3000 mg/kg diet. This was, however, a commonly observed change in old rats. Thus, tetramethrin did not affect the reproductive performance of male and female rats in two successive generations at up to 500 mg/kg diet [46].

7.7 Neurotoxicity - Mode of Action

Tetramethrin is classified as a Type I pyrethroid. The mode of action of pyrethroids in general is described in Appendix I.

In electrophysiological studies, tetramethrin produced repetitive discharges in housefly muscle and uncoupling in motor units [1, 32] and caused repetitive firing in cockroach cercal sensory nerves at a concentration of 3×10^{-13} mol/litre [8].

The effects of tetramethrin on the sodium channel gating mechanism were studied using the squid giant axons under voltage clamp conditions [27, 28]. Tetramethrin prolonged the falling phase of sodium current during depolarization and increased and prolonged the tail current associated with repolarization. The prolongation of the sodium current was due to the channel remaining open. The channel returned slowly to the resting state upon repolarization.

Analysis of the dose dependence of the two kinetic phases of tail current development suggests that the apparent dissociation constant for 1R,*trans*-tetramethrin depends on the conformational state of the channel. Thus, it can be concluded that tetramethrin binds to sodium channels and modifies the state of the channel in the resting, open, or inactivated state [28].

1R,*trans*-Tetramethrin markedly prolongs the open time of single sodium channels recorded by the gigaohm-seal voltage clamp technique in a membrane patch excised from the N1E-115 neuroblastoma cell. Single channel conductance is not altered by tetramethrin. The modification by tetramethrin occurs in an all-or-nothing manner in a population of sodium channels. The observed tetramethrin-induced modification of single sodium channels is compatible with previous sodium current data from axons [78].

Tetramethrin greatly prolongs the sodium current during step depolarization and the sodium tail current associated with step repolarization of the squid axon membrane. Non-linear current-voltage relationships for the sodium tail current were analyzed to assess the open sodium channel properties, which included the permeation of various cations, calcium block, and cation selectivity. Tetramethrin had no effect on any of these properties. It was concluded that tetramethrin modifies the sodium channel gating mechanism without affecting the pore properties [79].

8. EFFECTS ON HUMANS

Although tetramethrin has been used for many years, no adverse effects and no cases of human poisoning have been reported in the published literature.

In a semi-closed patch test, an aqueous emulsion containing 1.0% tetramethrin was applied to the skin of 200 human volunteers (aged 15-80, both male and female), using cotton gauze, for 4 days. After 2 weeks, an additional application was made in a same manner. Dermatological examination showed that tetramethrin is neither a primary irritant nor a human skin sensitizer [73].

9. PREVIOUS EVALUATION BY INTERNATIONAL BODIES

In the WHO Recommended Classification of Pesticides by Hazard, technical tetramethrin is classified as unlikely to present an acute hazard in normal use [75].

REFERENCES

1. ADAMS, M.E. & MILLER, T.A. (1980) Neurophysiological correlation of pyrethroid and DDT-type insecticide poisoning in the housefly *Musca domestica L.* In: *Insect neurobiology and pesticide action (Neutox 79)*, London, Society of Chemical Industry, pp. 431-439.

2. DING, C., YU, Y., ZHANG, J., CAI, Z., & CHAN, X. (1985) Genotoxic effects of tetramethrin on cultured mammalian cells and *Salmonella typhimurium. Zhejiang Yike Daxue Xuebao*, **14**(1): 1-4.

3. ELLIOTT, M. (1977) *Synthetic pyrethroids*, Washington, DC, American Chemical Society, p. 229 (ACS Symposium Series 42).

4. EVANS, M.H. (1976) End-plate potentials in frog muscle exposed to a synthetic pyrethroid *Pestic. Biochem. Physiol.*, **6**: 547-550.

5. FAO (1982) *Second Government Consultation on International Harmonization of Pesticide Registration Requirements, Rome, 11-15 October 1982*, Rome, Food and Agriculture Organization of the United Nations.

6. FLANNIGAN, S.A. & TUCKER, S.B. (1985) Variation in cutaneous sensation between synthetic pyrethroid insecticides. *Contact Dermatitis*, **13**: 140-147.

7. GAMMON, D.W. & CASIDA, J.E. (1983) Pyrethroids of the most potent class antagonize GABA action at the crayfish neuromuscular junction. *Neurosci. Lett.*, **40**: 163-168.

8. GAMMON, D.W., BROWN, M.A., & CASIDA, J.E. (1981) Two classes of pyrethroid action in the cockroach. *Pestic. Biochem. Physiol.*, **15**: 181-191.

9. GAMMON, D.W., LAWRENCE, L.J., & CASIDA, J.E. (1982) Pyrethroid toxicology: Protective effects of diazepam and phenobarbital in the mouse and the cockroach. *Toxicol. appl. Pharmacol.*, **66**: 290-296.

10. GLICKMAN, A.H. & CASIDA, J.E. (1982) Species and structural variations affecting pyrethroid neurotoxicity. *Neurobehav. Toxicol. Teratol.*, **4**:(6) 793-799.

11. HARA, S., SUZUKI, T., & MIYAMOTO, J. (1980a) *Primary eye and skin irritation tests of Neopynamin Forte® technical in rabbits* (Technical Report No. IT-00-0073) (Submitted to WHO by Sumitomo Chemical Co.).

12. HARA, S., SUZUKI, T., & MIYAMOTO, J. (1980b) *Skin sensitization test of Neopynamin Forte® technical in guinea-pigs* (Technical Report No. IT-00-0082) (Submitted to WHO by Sumitomo Chemical Co.).

13. HARA, M., SUZUKI, H., & MIYAMOTO, J. (1981) *In vivo chromosomal aberration test of Neopynamin Forte® on bone marrow cells of mice* (Technical Report No. 81042) (Submitted to WHO by Sumitomo Chemical Co.).

14. HARTLEY, D., KIDD, H., & KENNEDY, J.M. (1987) *Agrochemicals Handbook*, 2nd ed., Nottingham, United Kingdom, Royal Society of Chemistry.

15. HAYASHI, A. (1977) [How to use insecticides safely.] *Bo-satsu-kyo News*, **1**: 6-11 (in Japanese).

16. HIROMORI, T., HOSOKAWA, S., OKUNO, Y., SEKI, T., SUZUKI, T., & MIYAMOTO, J. (1982) [Mammalian toxicity of d-isomer of phthalthrin (Neopynamin Forte).] *Pharmacometrics*, **24**: 179-201 (in Japanese).

17. KADOTA, T., KOHDA, H., & MIYAMOTO, J. (1977) *Acute oral and dermal toxicities of Neopynamin in mice and rats* (Technical Report No. IT-70-0003) (Submitted to WHO by Sumitomo Chemical Co.).

18. KANEKO, H., OHKAWA, H., & MIYAMOTO, J. (1981) Metabolism of tetramethrin isomers in rats. *J. Pestic. Sci.*, **6**: 425-435.

19. KATO, T., UEDA, K., & FUJIMOTO, K. (1964) New insecticidally active chrysanthemates. *Agric. biol. Chem.*, **28**: 914-915.

20. KATO, T., SUZUKI, T., SAKO, H., OKUNO, Y., & MIYAMOTO, J. (1987) *Acute dermal toxicity of Neopynamin in rabbits* (Technical Report No. IT-70-0207) Submitted to WHO by Sumitomo Chemical Co.).

21. KAWAMOTO, M., HARA, M., KOGISO, S., YOSHITAKE, A., & YAMADA, H. (1988) *In vitro unscheduled DNA synthesis (UDS) assay of Neopynamin in rat hepatocytes* (Technical Report No. IT-80-0213) (Submitted to WHO by Sumitomo Chemical Co.).

22. KISHIDA, F., SUZUKI, H., & MIYAMOTO, J. (1981) *Mutagenicity test of Neopynamin Forte® in bacterial system* (Technical Report No. IT-00-0101) (Submitted to WHO by Sumitomo Chemical Co.).

23. LAWRENCE, L.J. & CASIDA, J.E. (1982) Pyrethroid toxicology: mouse intracerebral structure-toxicity relationship. *Pestic. Biochem. Physiol.*, **18**: 9-14.

24. LAWRENCE, L.J. & CASIDA, J.E. (1983) Stereospecific action of pyrethroid insecticides on the gamma-aminobutyric acid receptor-ionophore complex. *Science*, **221**: 1399-1401.

25. LAWRENCE, L.J., GEE, K.W., & YAMAMURA, H.I. (1985) Interactions of pyrethroid insecticides with chloride ionophore-associated binding sites. *Neurotoxicology*, **6**: 87-98.

26. LEAHEY, J.P. (1985) *The pyrethroid insecticides*, London, Taylor & Francis Ltd., p. 440.

27. LUND, A.E. & NARAHASHI, T. (1981) Kinetics of sodium channel modification by the insecticide tetramethrin in squid axon membranes. *J. Pharmacol. exp. Ther.*, **219**: 464-473.

28. LUND, A.E. & NARAHASHI, T. (1982) Dose-dependent interaction of the pyrethroid isomers with sodium channels of squid axon membranes. *Neurotoxicology*, **3**: 11-24.

29. LUND, A.E. & NARAHASHI, T. (1983) Kinetics of sodium channel modification as the basis for the variation in the nerve membrane effects of pyrethroids and DDT analogs. *Pestic. Biochem. Physiol.*, **20**: 203-216.

30. MARTIN, H. & WORTHING, C.R. (1977) *The pesticide manual*, 5th ed., Croydon, British Crop Protection Council, p. 502.

31. MEISTER, R.T., BERG, G.L., SINE, C., MEISTER, S., & POPLYK, J. (1983) *Farm chemicals handbook. Section C. Pesticide dictionary*, Willoughby, Ohio, Meister Publishing Company, p. C232.

32. MILLER, T.A. & ADAMS, M.E. (1977) Central vs peripheral action of pyrethroids on the housefly nervous system. In: Elliot, M., ed. *Synthetic pyrethroids*, Washington DC, American Chemical Society, pp. 98-115 (ACS Symposium Series No. 42).

33. MIYAMOTO, J. (1976) Degradation, metabolism and toxicity of synthetic pyrethroids. *Environ. Health Perspect.*, **14**: 15-28.

34. MIYAMOTO, J. (1981) The chemistry, metabolism and residue analysis of synthetic pyrethroids, *Pure appl. Chem.*, **53**: 1967-2022.

35. MIYAMOTO, J. & KEARNEY, P.C. (1983) *Pesticide chemistry, human welfare and the environment, Proceedings of the Fifth International Congress of Pesticide Chemistry, Kyoto, Japan, 29 August-4 September 1982*, Oxford, Pergamon Press, Vol. 1-4.

36. MIYAMOTO, J., SATO, Y., & YAMAMOTO, K. (1968) Biochemical studies on the mode of action of pyrethroidal insecticides. Part I. Metabolic fate of phthalthrin in mammals. *Agric. biol. Chem.*, **32**: 628-640.

37. MURANO, A. (1972) Determination of the optical isomers of insecticidal pyrethroids by gas-liquid chromatography. *Agric. biol. Chem.*, **36**: 2203-2211.

38. OKUNO, Y. (1982) *Exposure study with spraying of Neopynamin aerosol* (Technical Report No. IF-20-002) (Unpublished data submitted to WHO by Sumitomo Chemical Co.).

39. OKUNO, Y., KADOTA, T., & MIYAMOTO, J. (1976a) *Eye and skin irritation of Neopynamin in rabbits* (Technical Report No. IT-60-0014) (Submitted to WHO by Sumitomo Chemical Co.).

40. OKUNO, Y., KADOTA, T., & MIYAMOTO, J. (1976b) *Skin sensitization study of Neopynamin with guinea-pigs* (Technical Report No. IT-60-0013) (Submitted to WHO by Sumitomo Chemical Co.).

41. PANSHINA, T.N. & SASINOVICH, L.M. (1983) Toxicology of synthetic pyrethroids. *Khim. Selsk. Khoz.* **12**: 51-53.

42. PAPADOPOULOU-MOURKIDOU, E., IWATA, Y., & GUNTHER, F.A. (1981) Utilization of an infrared detector for selective liquid chromatographic analysis. 2. Formulation analysis of the pyrethroid insecticides allethrin, decamethrin, cypermethrin, phenothrin, and tetramethrin. *J. agric. food. Chem.*, **29**(6): 1105-1111.

43. PENCE, D.H., HAGEN, W.H., ALSAKER, R.D., DAWKINS, B.G., MARSHALL, P.M., & TACEY, R.L. (1981a) *Subchronic toxicity study in dogs. Neopynamin Final Report,* Vienna, Virginia, Hazleton Laboratories Inc. (Technical Report No. IT-11-0098) (Submitted to WHO by Sumitomo Chemical Co.).

44. PENCE, D.H., SEROTA, D.G., ALSAKER, R.D., BANAS, D.A., & KUNDZINS, W. (1981b) *Chronic toxicity study in rats. Neopynamin Technical Final Report*, Vienna, Virginia, Hazleton Laboratories, Inc. (Technical Report No. IT-11-0097) (Submitted to WHO by Sumitomo Chemical Co.).

45. PENCE, D.H., COX, R.H., DUDECK, L.E., ALSAKER, R.D., JONES, S.R., PARKER, G.A., HEPNER, K.E., & ZOETIS, T. (1986a) *Combined chronic toxicity and oncogenicity study in mice. Neopynamin Final Report,* Vienna, Virginia, Hazleton Laboratories, Inc. (Technical Report No. IT-61-0193) (Submitted to WHO by Sumitomo Chemical Co.).

46. PENCE, D.H., WOLFE, G.W., KULWICH, B.A., HEPNER, K.E., & SNYDER, F.G. (1986b) *Two-generation reproduction study in rats. Neopynamin Forte® Final Report,* Hazleton Laboratories, Inc. (Technical Report No. IT-61-0201) (Submitted to WHO by Sumitomo Chemical Co.).

47. RUIGT, G.S.F. & VAN DEN BERCKEN, J. (1986) Action of pyrethroids on a nerve-muscle preparation of the clawed frog, *Xenopus laevis*. *Pestic. Biochem. Physiol.*, **25**: 176-187.

48. RUTTER, H.A., Jr (1974) *One-generation reproduction study in rats. Neopynamin Final Report,* Vienna, Virginia, Hazleton Laboratories, Inc. (Technical Report No. IT-01-0081) (Submitted to WHO by Sumitomo Chemical Co.).

49. RUTTER, H.A., Jr, NELSON, L.W., KUNDZINS, W., & MCHUGH (1974) *Two-year dietary administration in the rat. Neopynamin Final Report,* Vienna, Virginia, Hazleton Laboratories, Inc. (Technical Report No. IT-41-0024) (Submitted to WHO by Sumitomo Chemical Co.).

50. RUZO, L.O., SMITH, I.H., & CASIDA, J.E. (1982) Pyrethroid photochemistry: photooxidation reactions of the chrysanthemates, phenothrin and tetramethrin. *J. agric. food Chem.*, **30**: 110-115.

51. SATO, T. & NARAMA, K. (1980a) *Reproduction test of Neopynamin. Part 1: Fertility study in rats,* Shizuoka, Hamamatsu Seigiken Research (Technical Report No. IT-01-0075) (Submitted to WHO by Sumitomo Chemical Co.).

52. SATO, T. & NARAMA, K. (1980b) *Reproduction test of Neopynamin. Part 2: Teratology study in rats,* Shizuoka, Hamamatsu Seigiken Research (Technical Report No. IT-01-0076) (Submitted to WHO by Sumitomo Chemical Co.).

53. SATO, T. & NARAMA, K. (1980c) *Reproduction test of Neopynamin. Part 3: Teratology study in rabbits*, Shizuoka, Hamamatsu Seigiken Research (Technical Report No. IT-01-0077) (Submitted to WHO by Sumitomo Chemical Co.).

54. SATO, T., TAGAWA, G., & NARAMA, K. (1980) *Reproduction test of Neopynamin. Part 4: Perinatal and postnatal study in rats*, Shizuoka, Hamamatsu Seigiken Research (Technical Report No. IT-01-0078) (Submitted to WHO by Sumitomo Chemical Co.).

55. SMITH, I.H., WOOD, E.J., & CASIDA, J.E. (1982) Glutathione conjugate of the pyrethroid tetramethrin. *J. agric. food Chem.*, **30**: 598-600.

56. SUZUKI, H. & MIYAMOTO, J. (1977) *Studies on mutagenicity of Neopynamin with bacterial systems* (Technical Report No. IT-70-0023) (Submitted to WHO by Sumitomo Chemical Co.).

57. SUZUKI, T. & MIYAMOTO, J. (1974) Metabolism of tetramethrin in houseflies and rats *in vitro*. *Pestic. Biochem. Physiol.*, **4**: 86-97.

58. SUZUKI, T., KOHDA, H., MISAKI, Y., OKUNO, Y., KOYAMA, Y., & MIYAMOTO, J. (1980) *Acute and subacute inhalation toxicity studies of Neopynamin Forte in rats* (Technical Report No. IT-10-0144) (Submitted to WHO by Sumitomo Chemical Co.).

59. TANAKA, H., TAKADA, S., ISEKI, M., SANO, R., AIHARA, H., KURODA, H., MAEBO, Y., MOTOYOSHI, I., & WAKAI, Y. (1967) Toxicological studies of various insecticides to mammalia. 2. On the acute and chronic toxicity of pyrethroid insecticide phthalthrin to albino rat or guinea-pig. *Med. J. Osaka City Univ.*, **16**: 509-517.

60. UEDA, K., GAUGHAN, L.C., & CASIDA, J E. (1975) Metabolism of (+)-trans- and (+)-cis-resmethrin in rats. *J. agric. food Chem.*, **23**: 106-115.

61. UNO, M., OKADA, T., OHMAE, T., TERADA, I., & TANIGAWA, K. (1982) [Determination of pyrethroid insecticides by dual-wavelength densitometry.] *Shokuhin Eiseigaku Zasshi*, **23**: 191-195 (in Japanese).

62. VAN DEN BERCKEN, J. (1977) The action of allethrin on the peripheral nervous system of the frog. *Pestic. Sci.*, **8**: 692-699.

63. VAN DEN BERCKEN, J. & VIJVERBERG, H.P.M. (1980) Voltage clamp studies on the effects of allethrin and DDT on the sodium channels in frog myelinated nerve membrane. In: *Insect neurobiology and pesticide action*, London, Society of Chemical Industry, pp. 79-85.

64. VAN DEN BERCKEN, J., AKKERMANS, L.M.A., & VAN DER ZALM, J.M. (1973) DDT-like action of allethrin in the sensory nervous system of *Xenopus laevis*. *Eur. J. Pharmacol.*, **21**: 95-106.

65. VAN DEN BERCKEN, J., KROESE, A.B.A., & AKKERMANS, L.M.A. (1979) Effect of insecticides on the sensory nervous system. In: Narahashi, T., ed. *Neurotoxicology of insecticides and phermones*, New York, London, Plenum Press, pp. 183-210.

66. VERSCHOYLE, R.D. & ALDRIDGE, W.N. (1980) Structure-activity relationship of some pyrethroids in rats. *Arch. Toxicol.*, **45**: 325-329.

67. VIJVERBERG, H.P.M. & VAN DEN BERCKEN, J. (1979) Frequency dependent effects of the pyrethroid insecticide decamethrin in frog myelinated nerve fibres. *Eur. J. Pharmacol.*, **58**: 501-504.

68. VIJVERBERG, H.P.M. & VAN DEN BERCKEN, J. (1982) Action of pyrethroid insecticides on the vertebrate nervous system. *Neuropathol. appl. Neurobiol.*, **8**: 421-440.

69. VIJVERBERG, H.P.M., RUIGT, G.S.F., & VAN DEN BERCKEN, J. (1982a) Structure-related effects of pyrethroid insecticides on the lateral-line sense organ and on peripheral nerves of the clawed frog, *Xenopus laevis*. *Pestic. Biochem. Physiol.*, **18**: 315-324.

70. VIJVERBERG, H.P.M., VAN DER ZALM, J.M., & VAN DEN BERCKEN, J. (1982b) Similar mode of action of pyrethroids and DDT on sodium channel gating in myelinated nerves. *Nature (Lond.)*, **295**: 601-603.

71. VIJVERBERG, H.P.M., VAN DER ZALM, J.M., VAN KLEEF, R.G.D.M., & VAN DEN BERCKEN, J. (1983) Temperature and structure-dependent interaction of pyrethroids with the sodium channels in frog node of Ranvier. *Biochim. Biophys. Acta*, **728**: 73-82.

72. WEIR, R.J. & CREWS, L.M. (1966) *Three month dietary administration to dogs of Neopynamin - final report* (Technical Report No. IT-61-0011) (Submitted to WHO by Sumitomo Chemical Co.).

73. WEIR, R.J. & OSBOURN, R.A. (1966) Report of human patch test on coded substance : 2301 D-61-1, Vienna, Virginia, Hazleton Laboratories, Inc. (Technical Report No. IT-61-0008) (Submitted to WHO by Sumitomo Chemical Co.).

74. WHO (1979) WHO Technical Report Series, No. 634 (Safe use of pesticides. Third Report of the WHO Expert Committee on Vector Biology and Control), pp. 18-23.

75. WHO (1988) *The WHO recommended classification of pesticides by hazard and guidelines to classification 1988/89*, Geneva, World Health Organization (Unpublished report VBC/88.953).

76. WORTHING, C.R. & WALKER, S.B. (1983) *The pesticide manual*, 7th ed., Croydon, British Crop Protection Council, p. 520.

77. WOUTERS, W. & VAN DEN BERCKEN, J. (1978) Action of pyrethroids. *Gen. Pharmacol.*, **9**: 387-398.

78. YAMAMOTO, D., QUANDT, F.N., & NARAHASHI, T. (1983) Modification of single sodium channels by the insecticide tetramethrin. *Brain Res*. **274**: 344-349.

79. YAMAMOTO, D., YEH, J.Z., & NARAHASHI, T. (1986) Ion permeation and selectivity of squid axon sodium channels modified by tetramethrin. *Brain Res.*, **372**: 193-197.

80. YOSHITAKE, A., KOGISO, S., HARA, M., & MIYAMOTO, J. (1986) *In vivo chromosomal aberration test of Neopynamin in mouse bone marrow cells* (Technical Report No. IT-60-0197) (Submitted to WHO by Sumitomo Chemical Co.).

81. YOSHITAKE, A., KOGISO, S., YAMADA, F., HARA, M., & MIYAMOTO, J. (1987) *Reverse mutation test of Neopynamin in Salmonella typhimurium and Escherichia coli* (Technical Report No. IT-70-0205) (Submitted to WHO by Sumitomo Chemical Co.).

APPENDIX 1

On the basis of electrophysiological studies with peripheral nerve preparations of frogs (*Xenopus laevis, Rana temporaria*, and *Rana esculenta*), it is possible to distinguish between 2 classes of pyrethroid insecticides: (Type I and Type II). A similar distinction between these 2 classes of pyrethroids has been made on the basis of the symptoms of toxicity in mammals and insects [10, 23, 65, 66, 74]. The same distinction was found in studies on cockroaches [8].

Based on the binding assay on the gamma-aminobutyric acid (GABA) receptor-ionophore complex, synthetic pyrethroids can also be classified into two types: the α-cyano-3-phenoxybenzyl pyrethroids and the non-cyano pyrethroids [7, 9, 24, 25].

Pyrethroids that do not contain an α-cyano group (allethrin, d-phenothrin, permethrin, tetramethrin, cismethrin, and bioresmethrin) (Type I: T-syndrome)

The pyrethroids that do not contain an α-cyano group give rise to pronounced repetitive activity in sense organs and in sensory nerve fibres [64]. At room temperature, this repetitive activity usually consists of trains of 3-10 impulses and occasionally up to 25 impulses. Train duration is between 10 and 5 milliseconds.

These compounds also induce pronounced repetitive firing of the presynaptic motor nerve terminal in the neuromuscular junction [62]. There was no significant effect of the insecticide on neurotransmitter release or on the sensitivity of the subsynaptic membrane, nor on the muscle fibre membrane. Presynaptic repetitive firing was also observed in the sympathetic ganglion treated with these pyrethroids.

In the lateral-line sense organ and in the motor nerve terminal, but not in the cutaneous touch receptor or in sensory nerve fibres, the pyrethroid-induced repetitive activity increases dramatically as the temperature is lowered, and a decrease of 5 °C in temperature may cause a more than 3-fold increase in the number of repetitive impulses per train. This effect is easily reversed by raising the temperature. The origin of this "negative temperature coefficient" is not clear [71].

Synthetic pyrethroids act directly on the axon through interference with the sodium channel gating mechanism that underlies the generation and conduction of each nerve impulse. The transitional state of the sodium channel is controlled by 2 separately acting gating mechanisms, referred to as the activation gate and the inactivation gate. Since pyrethroids only appear to affect the sodium current during depolarization, the rapid opening of the activation gate and the slow closing of the inactivation gate proceed normally. However, once the sodium channel is open, the activation gate is restrained in the open position by the pyrethroid molecule. While all pyrethroids have essentially the same basic mechanism of action, however, the rate of relaxation differs substantially for the various pyrethroids [6].

In the isolated node of Ranvier, allethrin causes prolongation of the transient increase in sodium permeability of the nerve membrane during excitation [63]. Evidence so far available indicates that allethrin selectively slows down the closing of the activation gate of a fraction of the sodium channels that open during depolarization of the membrane. The time constant of closing of the activation gate in the allethrin-affected channels is about 100 milliseconds compared with less than 100 microseconds in the normal sodium channel, i.e., it is slowed down by a factor of more than 100. This results in a marked prolongation of the sodium current across the nerve membrane during excitation, and this prolonged sodium current is directly responsible for the repetitive activity induced by allethrin [71].

The effects of cismethrin on synaptic transmission in the frog neuromuscular junction, as reported by Evans [4], are almost identical to those of allethrin, i.e., presynaptic repetitive firing, and no significant effects on transmitter release or on the subsynaptic membrane.

Interestingly, the action of these pyrethroids closely resembles that of the insecticide DDT in the peripheral nervous system of the frog. DDT also causes pronounced repetitive activity in sense organs, in sensory nerve fibres, and in motor nerve terminals, due to a prolongation of the transient increase in sodium permeability of the nerve membrane during excitation. Recently, it was demonstrated that allethrin and DDT have essentially the same effect on sodium channels in frog myelinated nerve membrane. Both compounds slow down the rate of closing of a fraction of the sodium channels that open on depolarization of the membrane [64, 65, 70].

In the electrophysiological experiments using giant axons of crayfish, the type I pyrethroids and DDT analogues retain sodium channels in a modified open state only intermittently, cause large depolarizing after-potentials, and evoke repetitive firing with minimal effect on the resting potential [29].

These results strongly suggest that permethrin and cismethrin, like allethrin, primarily affect the sodium channels in the nerve membrane and cause a prolongation of the transient increase in sodium permeability of the membrane during excitation.

The effects of pyrethroids on end-plate and muscle action potentials were studied in the pectoralis nerve-muscle preparation of the clawed frog (*Xenopus laevis).* Type I pyrethroids (allethrin, cismethrin, bioresmethrin, and 1R, *cis*-phenothrin) caused moderate presynaptic repetitive activity, resulting in the occurrence of multiple end-plate potentials [47].

Pyrethroids with an α-cyano group on the 3-phenoxybenzyl alcohol (deltamethrin, cyhalothrin, lambda-cyhalothrin, cypermethrin, fenvalerate, and fenpropanate) (Type II: CS-syndrome)

The pyrethroids with an α-cyano group cause an intense repetitive activity in the lateral line organ in the form of long-lasting trains of impulses [69]. Such a train may last for up to 1 min and contains thousands of impulses. The duration of the trains and the number of impulses per train increase markedly on lowering the temperature. Cypermethrin does not cause repetitive activity in myelinated nerve fibres. Instead, this pyrethroid causes a frequency-dependent depression of the nervous impulse, brought about by a progressive depolarization of the nerve membrane as a result of the summation of depolarizing after-potentials during train stimulation [67, 71].

In the isolated node of Ranvier, cypermethrin, like allethrin, specifically affects the sodium channels of the nerve membrane and causes a long-lasting prolongation of the transient increase in sodium permeability during excitation, presumably by slowing down the closing of the activation gate of the sodium channel [67, 71]. The time constant of closing of the activation gate in the cypermethrin-affected channels is prolonged to more than 100 milliseconds. Apparently, the amplitude of the prolonged sodium current after cypermethrin is too small to induce repetitive activity in nerve fibres, but is sufficient to cause the long-lasting repetitive firing in the lateral-line sense organ.

These results suggest that α-cyano pyrethroids primarily affect the sodium channels in the nerve membrane and cause a long-lasting prolongation of the transient increase in sodium permeability of the membrane during excitation.

In the electrophysiological experiments using giant axons of crayfish, the Type II pyrethroids retain sodium channels in a modified continuous open state persistently, depolarize the membrane, and block the action potential without causing repetitive firing [29].

Diazepam, which facilitates GABA reaction, delayed the onset of action of deltamethrin and fenvalerate, but not permethrin and allethrin, in both the mouse and cockroach. Possible mechanisms of the Type II pyrethroid syndrome include action at the GABA receptor complex or a closely linked class of neuroreceptor [9].

The Type II syndrome of intracerebrally administered pyrethroids closely approximates that of the convulsant picrotoxin (PTX). Deltamethrin inhibits the binding of [^{3}H]-dihydropicrotoxin to rat brain synaptic membranes, whereas the non-toxic R epimer of deltamethrin is inactive. These findings suggest a possible relation between the Type II pyrethroid action and the GABA receptor complex. The stereospecific correlation between the toxicity of Type II pyrethroids and their potency to inhibit the [^{35}S]-TBPS binding was established using a radioligand, [^{35}S]-*t*-butylbicyclophosphorothionate [^{35}S]-TBPS. Studies with 37 pyrethroids revealed an absolute correlation, without any false positive or negative, between mouse intracerebral toxicity and *in vitro* inhibition: all toxic cyano compounds including deltamethrin, 1R,*cis*-cypermethrin, 1R,*trans*-cypermethrin, and [2S, αS]-fenvalerate were inhibitors, but their non-toxic stereoisomers were not; non-cyano pyrethroids were much less potent or were inactive [24].

In the [^{35}S]-TBPS and [^{3}H]-Ro 5-4864 (a convulsant benzodiazepine radioligand) binding assay, the inhibitory potencies of pyrethroids were closely related to their mammalian toxicities. The most toxic pyrethroids of Type II were the most potent inhibitors of [^{3}H]-Ro 5-4864 specific binding to rat brain membranes. The [^{3}H]-dihydropicrotoxin and [^{35}S]-TBPS binding studies with pyrethroids strongly indicated that Type II effects of pyrethroids are mediated, at least in part, through an interaction with a GABA-regulated chloride ionophore-associated binding site. Moreover, studies with [^{3}H]-Ro 5-4864 support this hypothesis and, in addition, indicate that the pyrethroid-binding site may be very closely related to the convulsant benzodiazepine site of action [25].

The Type II pyrethroids (deltamethrin, 1R, *cis*-cypermethrin and [2S,αS]-fenvalerate) increased the input resistance of crayfish claw opener muscle fibres bathed in GABA. In contrast, two non-insecticidal stereoisomers and Type I pyrethroids (permethrin, resmethrin, allethrin) were inactive. Therefore, cyanophenoxybenzyl pyrethroids appear to act on the GABA receptor-ionophore complex [7].

The effects of pyrethroids on end-plate and muscle action potentials were studied in the pectoralis nerve-muscle preparation of the clawed frog (*Xenopus laevis).* Type II pyrethroids (cypermethrin and deltamethrin) induced trains of repetitive muscle action potentials without presynaptic repetitive activity. However, an intermediate group of pyrethroids (1R-permethrin, cyphenothrin, and fenvalerate) caused both types of effect. Thus, in muscle or nerve membrane the pyrethroid induced repetitive activities due to a prolongation of the sodium current.

But no clear distinction was observed between non-cyano and α-cyano pyrethroids [47].

Appraisal

In summary, the results strongly suggest that the primary target site of pyrethroid insecticides in the vertebrate nervous system is the sodium channel in the nerve membrane. Pyrethroids without an α-cyano group (allethrin, d-phenothrin, permethrin, and cismethrin) cause a moderate prolongation of the transient increase in sodium permeability of the nerve membrane during excitation. This results in relatively short trains of repetitive nerve impulses in sense organs, sensory (afferent) nerve fibres, and, in effect, nerve terminals. On the other hand, the α-cyano pyrethroids cause a long-lasting prolongation of the transient increase in sodium permeability of the nerve membrane during excitation. This results in long-lasting trains of repetitive impulses in sense organs and a frequency-dependent depression of the nerve impulse in nerve fibres. The difference in effects between permethrin and cypermethrin, which have identical molecular structures except for the presence of an α-cyano group on the phenoxybenzyl alcohol, indicates that it is this α-cyano group that is responsible for the long-lasting prolongation of the sodium permeability.

Since the mechanisms responsible for nerve impulse generation and conduction are basically the same throughout the entire nervous system, pyrethroids may also induce repetitive activity in various parts of the brain. The difference in symptoms of poisoning by α-cyano pyrethroids, compared with the classical pyrethroids, is not necessarily due to an exclusive central site of action. It may be related to the long-lasting repetitive activity in sense organs and possibly in other parts of the nervous system, which, in a more advance state of poisoning, may be accompanied by a frequency-dependent depression of the nervous impulse.

Pyrethroids also cause pronounced repetitive activity and a prolongation of the transient increase in sodium permeability of the nerve membrane in insects and other invertebrates. Available information indicates that the sodium channel in the nerve membrane is also the most important target site of pyrethroids in the invertebrate nervous system [74, 77].

Because of the universal character of the processes underlying nerve excitability, the action of pyrethroids should not be considered restricted to particular animal species, or to a certain region of the nervous system. Although it has been established that sense organs and nerve endings are the most vulnerable to the action of pyrethroids, the ultimate lesion that causes death will depend on the animal species, environmental conditions, and on the chemical structure and physical characteristics of the pyrethroid molecule [68].

1. RESUME, EVALUATION, CONCLUSIONS ET RECOMMANDATIONS

1.1 Résumé et évaluation

1.1.1 Identité, propriétés physiques et chimiques, méthodes d'analyse

La tétraméthrine a été synthétisée pour la première fois en 1964 et commercialisée et en 1965. Sur la plan chimique, c'est un ester de l'acide chrysanthémique (acide diméthyl-2,2(diméthyl-2,2 vinyl)-3 cyclopropanecarboxylique et de l'alcool tétrahydro-3,4,5,6 phatlimidométhylique. Elle est constituée d'un mélange de quatre stéréoisomères [1R,trans], [1R,cis], [1S,trans] et [1S,cis]. Les stéréo-isomères qui entrent dans la composition des produits techniques sont à peu près dans la proportion de 4:1:4:1. De tous les isomères, c'est l'isomère [1R,trans] qui est le plus actif biologiquement; vient ensuite l'isomère 1R,cis]. On commercialise sous le nom de "Neo-pynamine Forte" (désignée dans la présente monographie sous le nom de 1R,*cis/trans*-tetraméthrine), un mélange des isomères [1R,cis] et [1R,trans] dans le proportion de 1:4.

La tétraméthrine de qualité technique est un solide incolore dont le point de fusion est de 60-80 °C. Sa densité est de 1,11 à 20 °C et sa tension de vapeur de 0,946 mPa (7,1 x 10^{-6} mm Hg) à 30 °C. Peu soluble dans l'eau (4,6 mg/litre à 30 °C), elle est en revanche soluble dans certains solvants organiques tels que l'hexane, le méthanol et le xylène. Elle est stable à la chaleur mais instable à la lumière et à l'air. L'isomère [1R,cis/trans] est un liquide visqueux de couleur jaune dont les autres propriétés physiques et les propriétés chimiques sont les mêmes que celles de la tétraméthrine.

Le dosage des résidus s'effectue par densitométrie à deux longueurs d'onde (370-230 nm). Pour l'analyse des produits techniques, on utilise la chromatographie en phase gazeuse avec détection par ionisation de flamme. Une analyse des différentes formulations peut s'effectuer au moyen d'un chromatographe en phase liquide à haute performance muni d'un détecteur infrarouge.

1.1.2 Production et usage

La production mondiale annuelle de tétraméthrine est évaluée à quelques centaines de tonnes. Elle est principalement utilisée pour la lutte contre les nuisibles à l'intérieur des habitations, sous forme d'aérosols, de concentrés émulsionnables ou de serpentins anti-moustiques. La tétraméthrine entre également dans la composition d'autres formulations insecticides additionnées ou non de synergisants.

1.1.3 Exposition humaine

L'exposition de la population dans son ensemble peut résulter de l'utilisation de ce produit pour la destruction des nuisibles dans les habitations. Lorsqu'on utilise la tétraméthrine conformément aux recommandations, sa concentration atmosphérique ainsi que celle de l'isomère 1R ne devraient pas dépasser 0,5 mg/m^3; par ailleurs le composé se dégrade rapidement. L'exposition de la population générale est donc vraisemblablement très faible. On n'utilise pas de tétraméthrine pour traiter les cultures vivrières.

1.1.4 Exposition et destinée dans l'environnement

Une fine pellicule de tétraméthrine exposée à la lumière solaire se dégrade rapidement. On a observé que les principales réactions photochimiques qui se produisaient au cours d'une exposition de 2 heures (conversion de 30%) étaient: une époxydation au niveau de la double liaison du radical isobuténylе, une oxydation en hydroxyméthyle, en aldéhyde et en acide carboxylique du groupe méthyle en position trans du groupement isobuténylе; enfin, une hydroperoxydation en hydroperoxyde allylique.

On ne connaît pas avec exactitude les concentrations exactes de tétraméthrine dans l'environnement, mais compte tenu de l'utilisation qui en est faite actuellement pour traiter les habitations et pourvu que le produit soit utilisé conformément aux recommandations, il est vraisemblable que l'exposition dans l'environnement devrait être très faible. La tétraméthrine se décompose rapidement en produits moins toxiques.

1.1.5 *Absorption, métabolisme, et excrétion*

Des rats à qui l'on avait administré par voie orale ou sous-cutanée de la tétraméthrine radio-marquée au niveau du reste acide ou du reste alcool ont rapidement absorbé, métabolisé et excrété le produit. L'excrétion s'effectue en 5 à 7 jours dans la proportion d'environ 95%, à peu près autant par la voie urinaire que par la voie fécale. Par ces deux voies, les résidus présents dans les tissus sont très faibles. La métabolisation s'effectue par les réactions suivantes: coupure de l'ester; élimination du groupe hydroxyméthyl du reste alcool; réduction de la double liaison 1-2 du reste alcool; oxydation du groupement méthyle de l'isobutényle au niveau du reste acide et en 2, 3 et 4 au niveau du reste alcool; conjugaison des acides et des alcools résultant avec l'acide glucuronique et enfin isomérisation cis/trans.

1.1.6 *Effets sur les êtres vivant dans leur milieu naturel*

On ne dispose que de très peu d'informations à ce sujet. La tétramethrine est extrêmement toxique pour les poissons, la valeur de la CL_{50} à 96-h pour deux espèces se situant respectivement à 19 et 21 μg/litre. Pour une troisième espèce, on a obtenu une CL_{50} à 48 heures de 200 μg/litre et la dose sans effet observable était de 50 μg/litre. Pour la daphnie, la dose sans effet observable est également de 50 μg/litre. La tétraméthrine est en revanche très peu toxique pour les oiseaux mais elle est toxique pour les abeilles. Cependant du fait que le produit est rapidement dégradé et dans la mesure où on ne l'utilise, conformément aux recommandations, que dans les habitations, il est peu probable qu'il puisse excercer des effets nocifs sur l'environnement.

1.1.7 *Effets sur les animaux d'expérience et sur les systèmes d'épreuve* in-vitro

La tétraméthrine a une faible toxicité aiguë par voie orale. La DL_{50} pour le rat est >5000 mg/kg, qu'il s'agisse du racémique ou de l'isomère (1R,cis/trans), tandis que pour la souris elle est d'environ 2000 mg/kg (racémique) et de 1060 mg/kg (1R,cis/trans). Chez le rat, la souris et le lapin la toxicité aiguë par voie percutanée est également faible; la DL_{50} chez le rat et la souris étant <5000 mg/kg et <2000 mg/kg chez le lapin (toutes les études portaient sur le racémique). Les études de toxicité aiguë par inhalation ont donné une CL_{50} chez le rat et la souris de 2500 mg/m^3 pour le racémique et >1180 mg/m^3 pour l'isomère (1R,cis/trans). Parmi les signes d'intoxication on a noté une hyperexcitabilité, des tremblements, de l'ataxie et une dépression (signes généraux observés dans l'ensemble des études de toxicité aiguë). Les souris se sont révélées un peu plus sensibles que les rats mais il n'y avait pas de différences de sensibilité entre mâles et femelles. Qu'ils s'agisse du racémique ou de l'isomère (1R,cis/trans), la tétraméthrine ne provoque pratiquement aucune irritation oculaire ou cutanée chez le lapin. En outre, ni l'un ni l'autre de ces produits n'exercent d'effet sensibilisateur chez le cobaye.

La tétraméthrine est un pyréthroïde du type I. Chez les mammifères ce sont les tremblements (syndrome-T) qui constituent le symptôme d'intoxication caractéristique.

Chez des rats ayant reçu de la tétraméthrine mêlée à leur nourriture à des concentrations allant jusqu'à 5000 mg/kg de nourriture pendant 91 jours, on a noté une réduction du gain de poids à la dose la plus forte. D'après les résultats d'études de 3 et 6 mois, au cours desquelles des rats ont reçu l'isomère 1R(cis/trans) dans leur nourriture à des doses allant de 25 mg/kg à 3000 mg/kg d'aliment, la dose sans effet observable était de 200 mg/kg de nourriture pour les mâles et de 300 mg/kg pour les femelles (parmi les anomalies observées, on notait une réduction du gain de poids et du poids final du corps ainsi que certains effets sur les reins et le foie). Les effets sur le foie résultent, semble-t-il, d'une réaction d'adaptation à la présence dans l'alimentation du véhicule utilisé, à savoir l'huile de maïs.

Une étude de 26 semaines sur des chiens a fait ressortir une dose sans effet observable de 1250 mg/kg de nourriture.

Des souris et des rats à qui l'on avait fait inhaler de la tétraméthrine en aérosol à une concentration de 200 mg/m^3, 3 à 4 heures par jour pendant des périodes allant jusqu'à quatre semaines, n'ont présenté aucune anomalie imputable à ce produit. Lors d'une autre étude de ce type, au cours de laquelle des rats ont été exposés à une brumisation (gouttelettes de 1,2-1,5 μm de diamètre) d'isomère (1R,cis/trans) dans du kérosène désodorisé à des concentrations allant jusqu'à 87 mg/m^3, trois heures par jour et sept jours par semaine pendant 28 jours, on a obtenu, pour la dose sans effet observable, une valeur de 49 mg/m^3. Les signes d'intoxication n'ont été observés qu'au cours de l'exposition.

Ni la tétraméthrine ni ses isomères (1R,cis/trans) ne se sont révélés mutagènes dans divers systèmes d'épreuve *in vivo* et *in vitro* utilisés pour étudier les mutations génétiques, les lésions et les réparations de l'ADN ainsi que les effets sur les chromosomes.

Trois études, dont deux chez le rat et une chez la souris ont été menées pendant 104 semaines afin d'étudier la cancérogénicité à long terme de la tétraméthrine. Les souris ont reçu de la tétraméthrine dans leur nourriture à des doses allant jusqu'à 1500 mg/kg de nourriture. Aucun effet oncogène n'a été observé. A partir de 60 mg/kg de nourriture on observait une réduction du poids de l'hypophyse, de la thyroïde et de la parathyroïde. Chez la souris, la dose sans effet général observable se situait à 12 mg/kg de nourriture. Quant aux rats, ils ont été exposés à de la tétraméthrine à des doses allant jusqu'à 5000 mg/kg de nourriture soit *in utero* soit au cours d'une période prolongée. Les deux études ont fait ressortir un gain de poids sensiblement moindre chez les animaux recevant 3000 mg de tétraméthrine par kg de nourriture ou davantage. En outre, à ces concentrations, on a observé une augmentation du poids du foie. Pour ce qui est des effets généraux, la dose sans effet observable se situait dans les deux études, à 1000 mg/kg de nourriture. A la dose de 3000 mg/kg de nourriture, l'incidence des tumeurs testiculaires à cellules de Leydig était supérieure à la valeur notée dans le groupe témoin et ce, pour les deux études. Les tumeurs à cellules de Leydig se produisent spontanément chez les rats âgés et leur incidence peut varier énormément dans les groupes témoins. On pense que cette tumeur est d'origine hormonale. Aucun signe de malignité et aucune tumeur de ce type n'ont été relevés chez les souris. On peut en conclure que cet effet oncogène, s'il existe réellement, ne peut être pris en considération pour ce qui concerne l'homme.

La tétraméthrine ne s'est révélée ni tératogène ni embryotoxique à des doses allant jusqu'à 1000 mg par kg de poids corporel chez les rats et jusqu'à 500 mg/kg chez des lapins (il s'agit des concentrations les plus fortes étudiées). Lors d'une étude de fécondité au cours de laquelle des rats ont reçu de la tétraméthrine à des doses allant jusqu'à 1000 mg/kg de poids corporel par jour, la dose sans effet observable sur la reproduction des parents et la croissance des foetus, se situait à 300 mg/kg de poids corporel par jour. Une étude de reproduction chez le rat, portant sur la période périnatale et sur la période post-natale, a permis de fixer à 100 mg/kg de poids corporel la dose quotidienne sans effet observable (la dose la plus forte administrée au cours de cette étude).

Lors d'une étude de reproduction portant sur une génération de rats, on a administré aux animaux 1000-6000 mg de tétraméthrine par kg de nourriture et constaté que la dose sans effet observable était de 1000 mg/kg. Selon une autre étude portant cette fois sur deux générations, au cours de laquelle les rats ont reçu de l'isomère (1R,cis/trans) à des doses allant de 100 à 3000 mg/kg, la dose sans effet observable était de 500 mg/kg de nourriture.

1.1.8 Effets sur l'homme

Bien que la tétraméthrine et son isomère 1R soient utilisées depuis des années, on ne signale aucun cas d'intoxication ou d'effets indésirables chez l'homme.

Rien n'indique que la tétraméthrine ou son isomère 1R puissent avoir des effets nocifs sur l'homme si on continue de les utiliser à faibles concentrations et seulement pour la destruction des nuisibles à l'intérieur des habitations.

1.2 Conclusions

a) Population générale: l'exposition de la population générale à la tétraméthrine, dans son utilisation actuelle, est vraisemblablement faible. Si ce produit est utilisé conformément aux recommandations, il ne présente probablement aucun risque.

b) L'exposition professionnelle: moyennant de bonnes méthodes de travail, l'application de mesures d'hygiène et avec quelques précautions, la tétraméthrine ne devrait pas présenter de danger pour les personnes qui y sont exposées de par leur profession.

c) Environnement: il est tout à fait improbable que la tétraméthrine ou ses produits de décomposition s'accumulent au point d'avoir des effets nocifs sur l'environnement.

1.3 Recommandations

Bien que la tétraméthrine et son isomère 1R soient utilisés depuis des années sans qu'on ait à déplorer d'effets nocifs chez l'homme, il est souhaitable que l'exposition humaine continue d'être surveillée.